ACUPUNCTURE

LOGIC

I0511048

ACUPUNCTURE
TREATMENT
ALGORITHMS

Michael J. Migliore, R.Ph., M.S., L.Ac.

© Copyright 2003 Michael J. Migliore. All rights reserved.

No part of this publication may be reproduced, stored in a retrieval system, or transmitted, in any form or by any means, electronic, mechanical, photocopying, recording, or otherwise, without the written prior permission of the author.

National Library of Canada Cataloguing in Publication

Migliore, Michael J.
      Acupuncture logic / Michael J. Migliore.
ISBN 1-55395-663-X
      1. Acupuncture. I. Title.
RM184.M43 2003   615.8'92   C2003-900286-1

TRAFFORD

This book was published *on-demand* in cooperation with Trafford Publishing. On-demand publishing is a unique process and service of making a book available for retail sale to the public taking advantage of on-demand manufacturing and Internet marketing. **On-demand publishing** includes promotions, retail sales, manufacturing, order fulfilment, accounting and collecting royalties on behalf of the author.

Suite 6E, 2333 Government St., Victoria, B.C. V8T 4P4, CANADA
Phone   250-383-6864   Toll-free 1-888-232-4444 (Canada & US)
Fax   250-383-6804   E-mail   sales@trafford.com
Web site www.trafford.com   TRAFFORD PUBLISHING IS A DIVISION OF TRAFFORD HOLDINGS LTD.
Trafford Catalogue #03-0026   www.trafford.com/robots/03-0026.html

10   9   8   7   6   5   4   3

NOTE

With respect to the nature of the material and information presented in this book, the author and publishers have to the best of their knowledge made every attempt to validate the accuracy of this publication. At the time of this publication, the information contained in this book is consistent with the standards of practice generally accepted in the acupuncture communities. The author and publishers disclaim any liability, loss, injury or damage incurred as a consequence, directly or indirectly, of the use and application of any of the contents of this book.

ABOUT THE AUTHOR

Michael J. Migliore is a licensed acupuncturist and a Diplomate in Acupuncture by the National Certification Commission of Acupuncture and Oriental Medicine. He is a registered pharmacist and former self-employed independent community pharmacy practitioner. The author is the founder and director of the Landmark Wellness Center, where he currently maintains a private acupuncture practice in New York City. He serves on the board of directors for the Acupuncture Society of New York as well as a not-for-profit home health care agency serving the five boroughs of New York City. Presently, he is an adjunct professor at the Pacific College of Oriental Medicine, NYC.

Dedicated
to my parents
and
their parents.

ACKNOWLEDGEMENTS

To my
teachers,
family,
friends,
and
patients,

and

to my
wife MaryAnn,
for
without her,
this book
would not be
possible.

MJM
Staten Island, New York
2002

PREFACE: How to use this Book

The information contained in this book, although familiar to many practitioners and students, is presented in a concise logistical format. This unique method of utilizing acupuncture treatment algorithms for differential diagnosis of disease states is logically systematic and useful both as an acupuncture treatment text and reference guide. The compilation of material is extracted from *Chinese Acupuncture and Moxibustion*, Foreign Language Press, Beijing. The disease states are listed alphabetically and are located at the top of the page. They are then subcategorized and differentiated according to their main manifestations. The acupuncture treatment points that are specific to the disease state are found next, followed by the tongue and pulse diagnosis. Located at the bottom of the page are acupuncture treatment points that are common to the various subdivisions of the disease states. It is often helpful to start at the bottom of the page, identifying common acupuncture treatment points to each subdivision (if there are any). This unique presentation of the material appears visually clear, uniform and easier to decipher and commit to memory. The appendix contains the disease states and acupuncture treatment points listed in a quick reference chart. This document will prove to be a valuable tool to both practitioner and student.

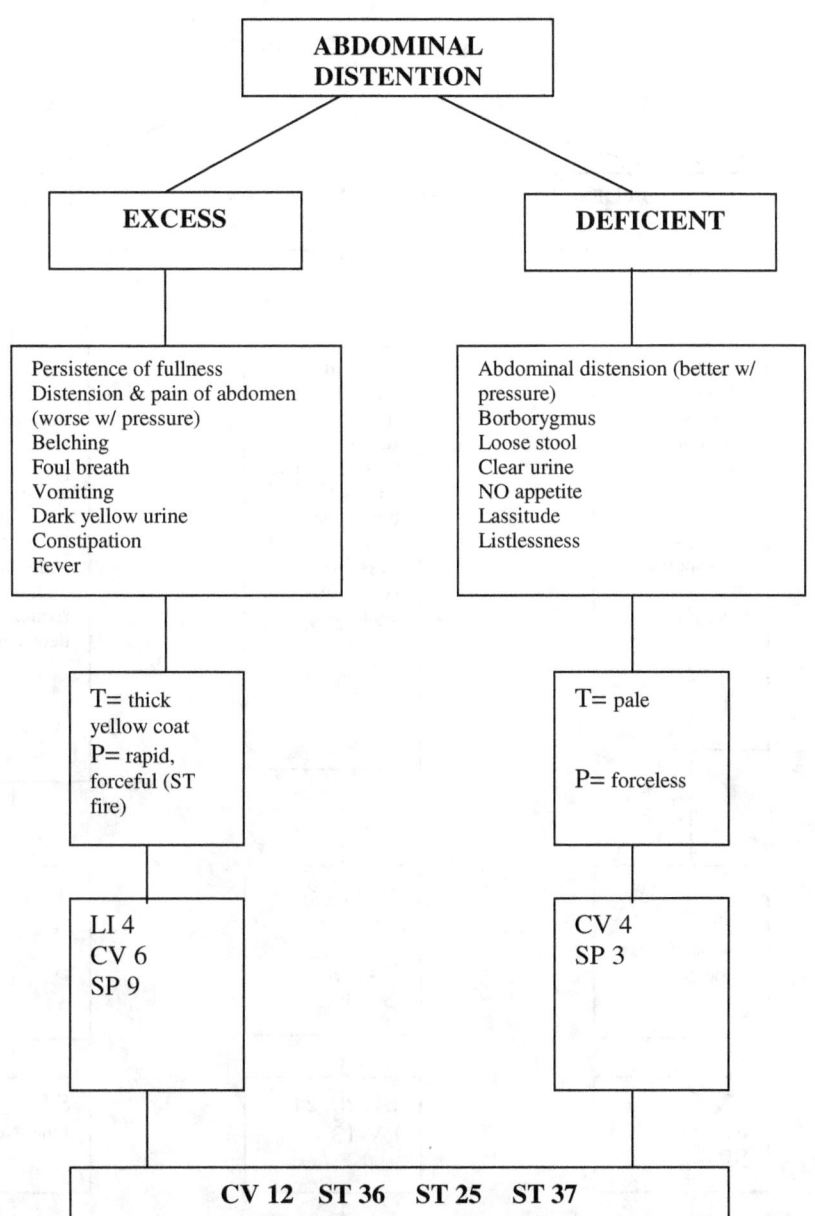

ABDOMINAL DISTENTION

EXCESS

DEFICIENT

Persistence of fullness
Distension & pain of abdomen
(worse w/ pressure)
Belching
Foul breath
Vomiting
Dark yellow urine
Constipation
Fever

Abdominal distension (better w/
pressure)
Borborygmus
Loose stool
Clear urine
NO appetite
Lassitude
Listlessness

T= thick
yellow coat
P= rapid,
forceful (ST
fire)

T= pale

P= forceless

LI 4
CV 6
SP 9

CV 4
SP 3

CV 12   ST 36   ST 25   ST 37

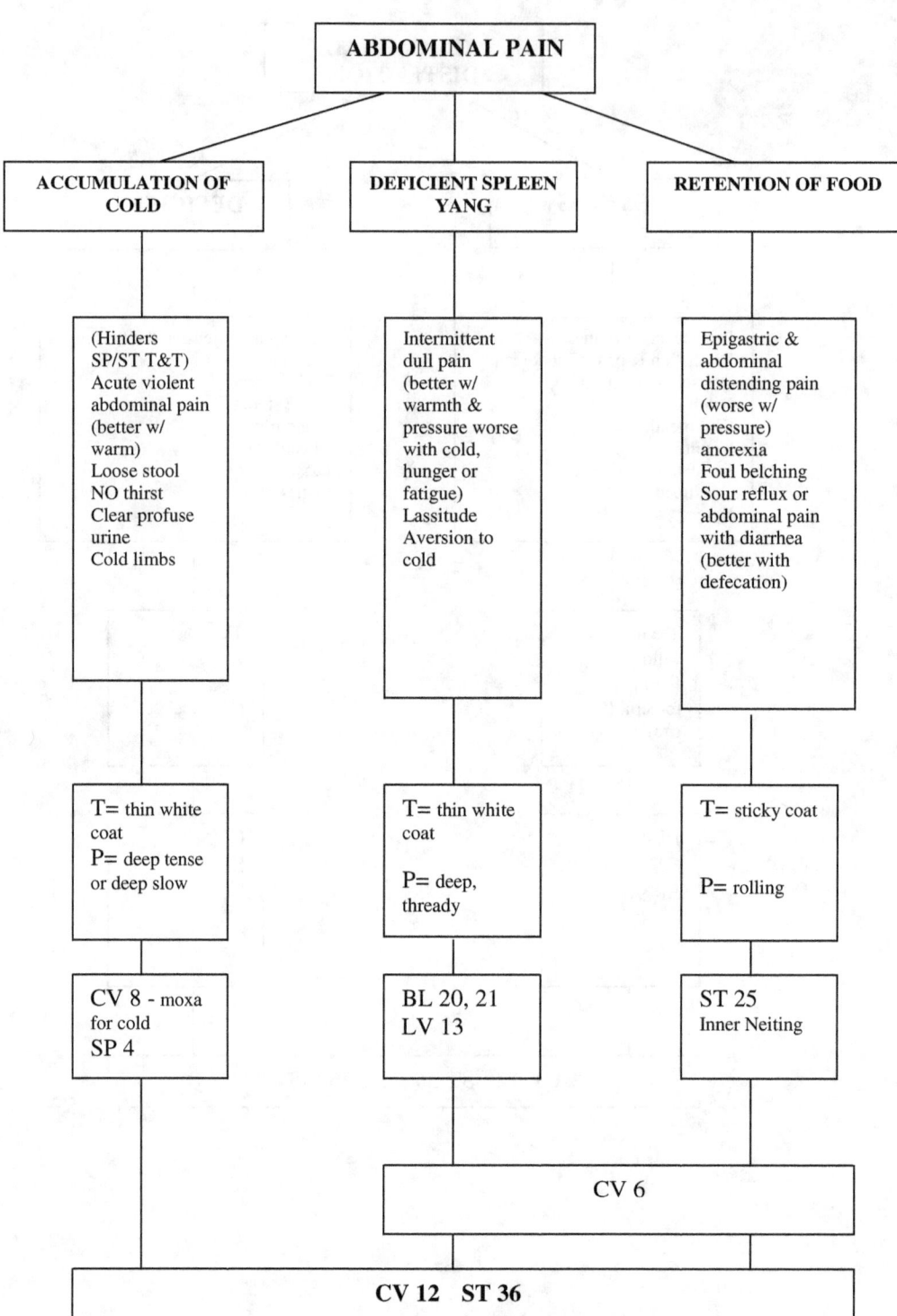

ABDOMINAL PAIN

ACCUMULATION OF COLD

(Hinders SP/ST T&T)
Acute violent abdominal pain (better w/ warm)
Loose stool
NO thirst
Clear profuse urine
Cold limbs

T= thin white coat
P= deep tense or deep slow

CV 8 - moxa for cold
SP 4

DEFICIENT SPLEEN YANG

Intermittent dull pain (better w/ warmth & pressure worse with cold, hunger or fatigue)
Lassitude
Aversion to cold

T= thin white coat

P= deep, thready

BL 20, 21
LV 13

RETENTION OF FOOD

Epigastric & abdominal distending pain (worse w/ pressure) anorexia
Foul belching
Sour reflux or abdominal pain with diarrhea (better with defecation)

T= sticky coat

P= rolling

ST 25
Inner Neiting

CV 6

CV 12   ST 36

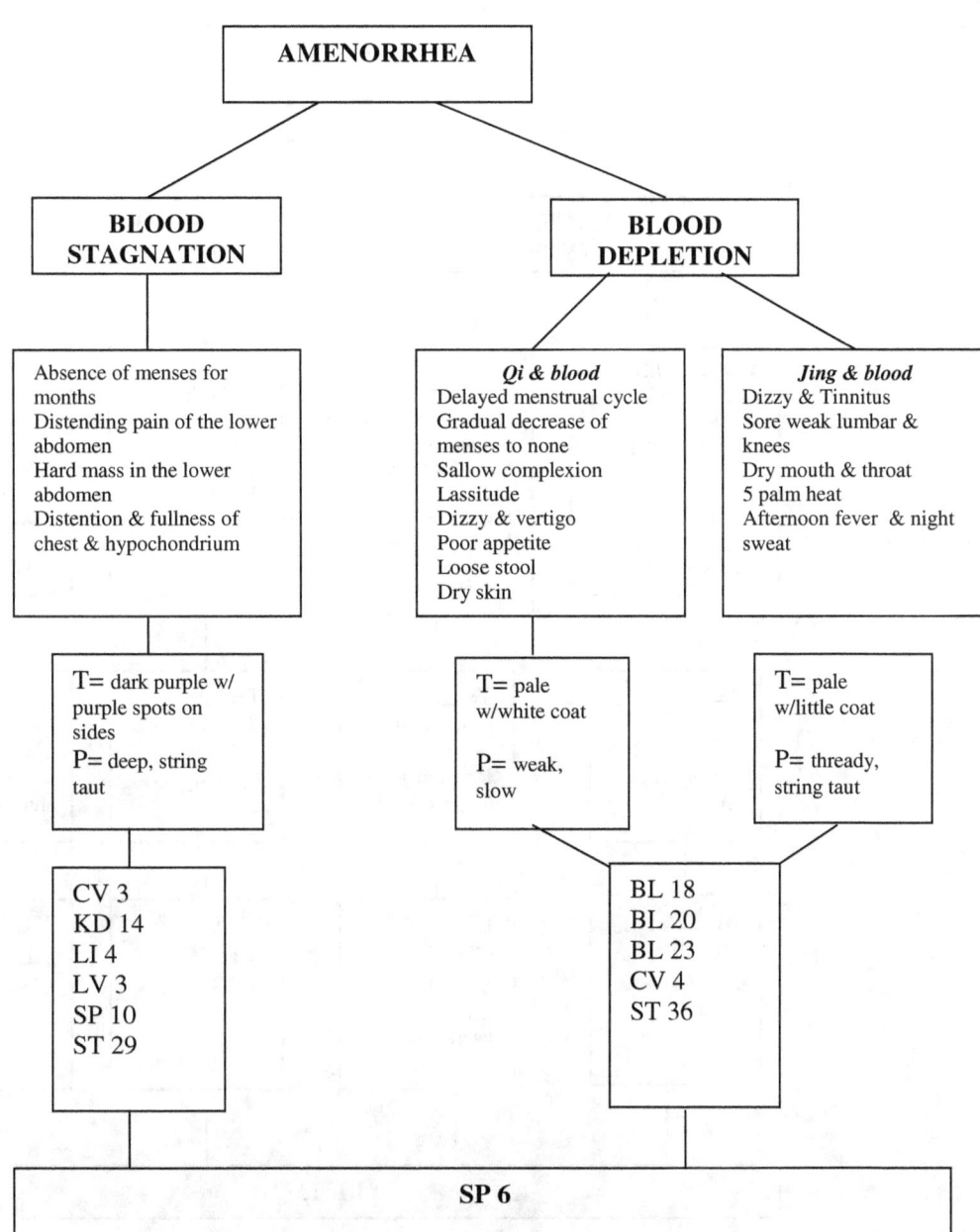

AMENORRHEA

BLOOD STAGNATION

BLOOD DEPLETION

Absence of menses for months
Distending pain of the lower abdomen
Hard mass in the lower abdomen
Distention & fullness of chest & hypochondrium

Qi & blood
Delayed menstrual cycle
Gradual decrease of menses to none
Sallow complexion
Lassitude
Dizzy & vertigo
Poor appetite
Loose stool
Dry skin

Jing & blood
Dizzy & Tinnitus
Sore weak lumbar & knees
Dry mouth & throat
5 palm heat
Afternoon fever & night sweat

T= dark purple w/ purple spots on sides

P= deep, string taut

T= pale w/white coat

P= weak, slow

T= pale w/little coat

P= thready, string taut

CV 3
KD 14
LI 4
LV 3
SP 10
ST 29

BL 18
BL 20
BL 23
CV 4
ST 36

SP 6

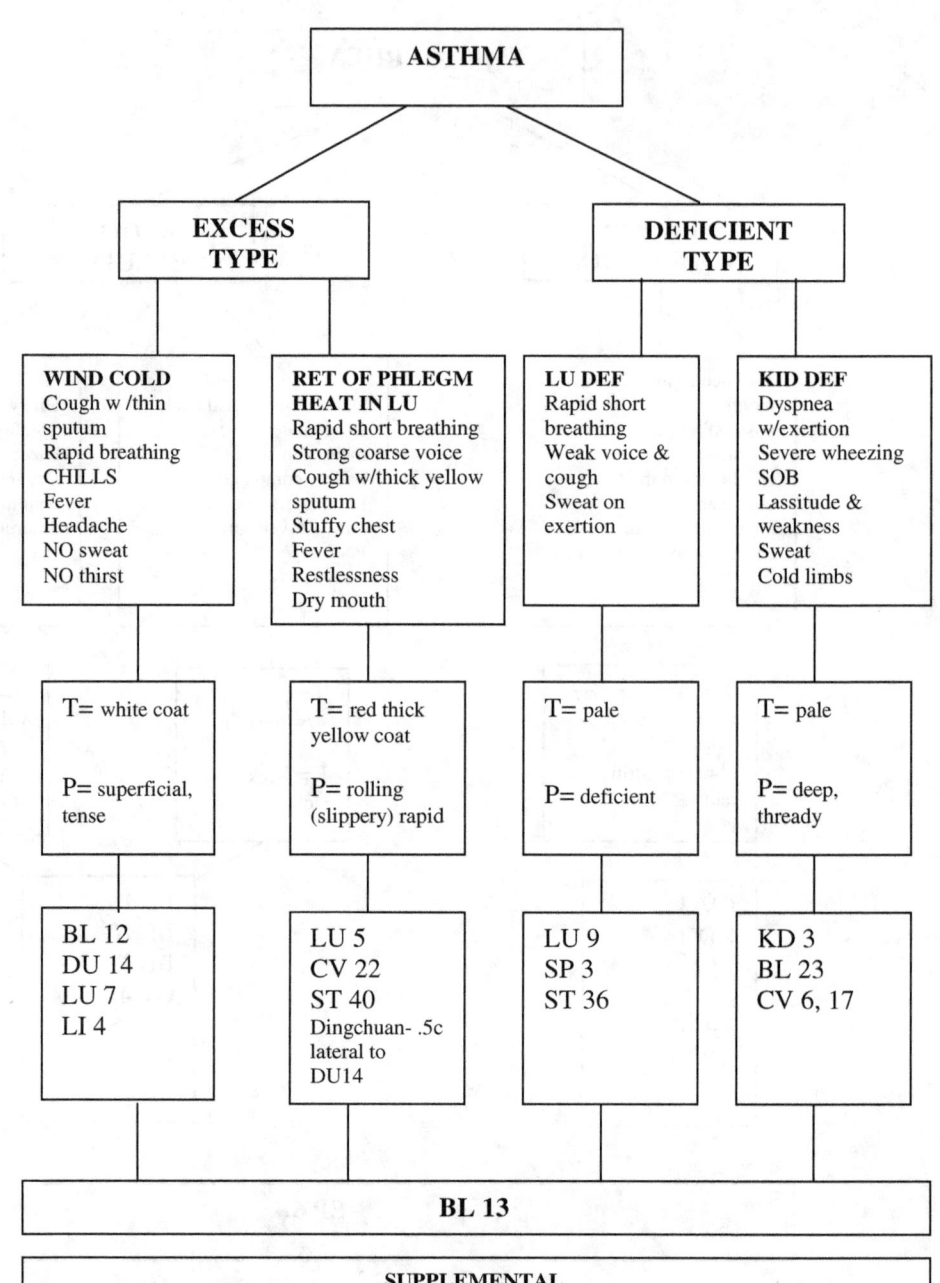

ASTHMA

EXCESS TYPE

DEFICIENT TYPE

WIND COLD
Cough w /thin sputum
Rapid breathing
CHILLS
Fever
Headache
NO sweat
NO thirst

RET OF PHLEGM HEAT IN LU
Rapid short breathing
Strong coarse voice
Cough w/thick yellow sputum
Stuffy chest
Fever
Restlessness
Dry mouth

LU DEF
Rapid short breathing
Weak voice & cough
Sweat on exertion

KID DEF
Dyspnea w/exertion
Severe wheezing
SOB
Lassitude & weakness
Sweat
Cold limbs

T= white coat

P= superficial, tense

T= red thick yellow coat

P= rolling (slippery) rapid

T= pale

P= deficient

T= pale

P= deep, thready

BL 12
DU 14
LU 7
LI 4

LU 5
CV 22
ST 40
Dingchuan- .5c lateral to DU14

LU 9
SP 3
ST 36

KD 3
BL 23
CV 6, 17

BL 13

SUPPLEMENTAL
Moxa DU 12 & BL 43 for chronic asthma   ----   Moxa CV12 & BL 20 for SP deficiency

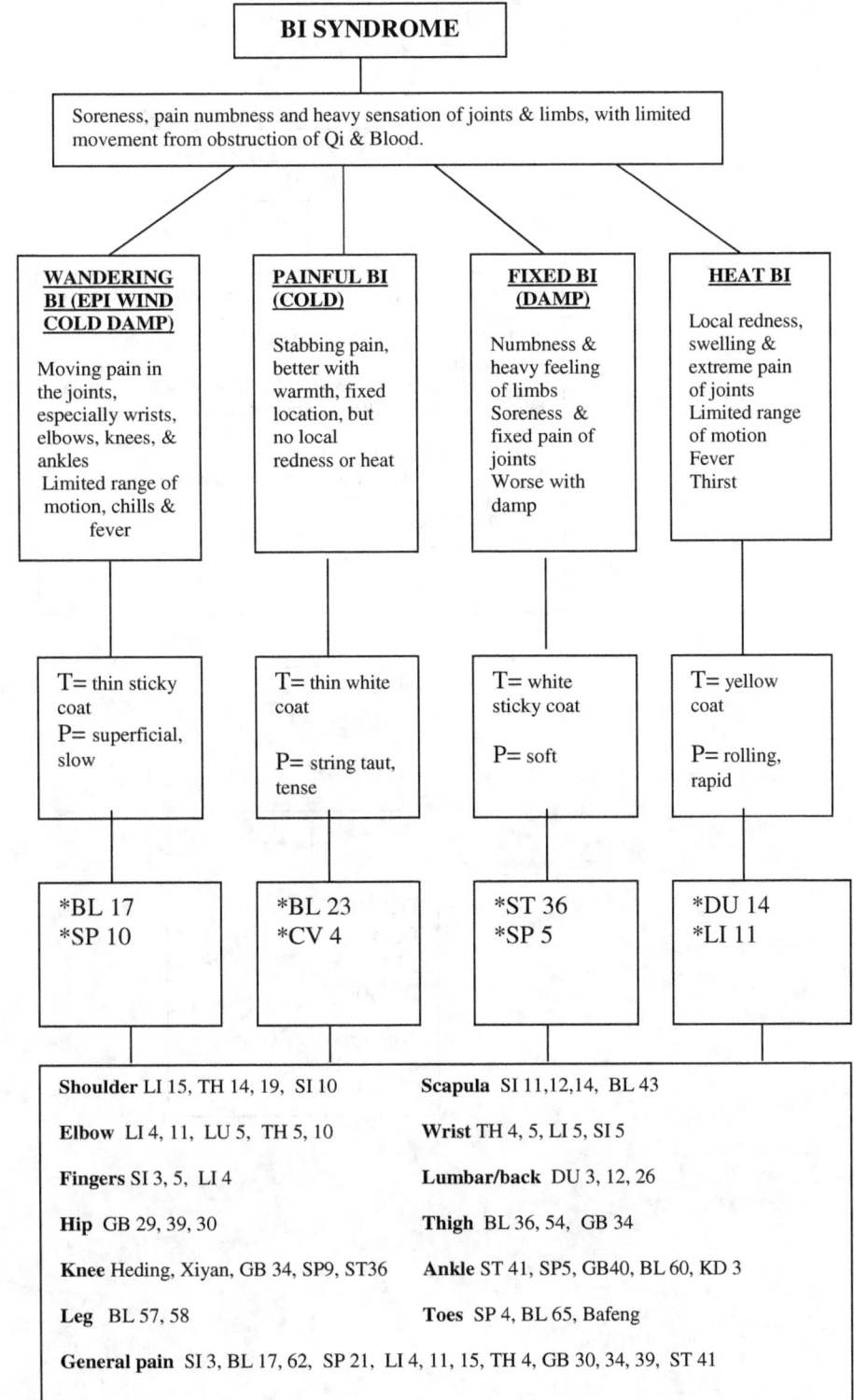

BI SYNDROME

Soreness, pain numbness and heavy sensation of joints & limbs, with limited movement from obstruction of Qi & Blood.

WANDERING BI (EPI WIND COLD DAMP)	PAINFUL BI (COLD)	FIXED BI (DAMP)	HEAT BI
Moving pain in the joints, especially wrists, elbows, knees, & ankles Limited range of motion, chills & fever	Stabbing pain, better with warmth, fixed location, but no local redness or heat	Numbness & heavy feeling of limbs Soreness & fixed pain of joints Worse with damp	Local redness, swelling & extreme pain of joints Limited range of motion Fever Thirst
T= thin sticky coat P= superficial, slow	T= thin white coat P= string taut, tense	T= white sticky coat P= soft	T= yellow coat P= rolling, rapid
*BL 17 *SP 10	*BL 23 *CV 4	*ST 36 *SP 5	*DU 14 *LI 11

Shoulder LI 15, TH 14, 19, SI 10   **Scapula** SI 11,12,14, BL 43

Elbow LI 4, 11, LU 5, TH 5, 10   **Wrist** TH 4, 5, LI 5, SI 5

Fingers SI 3, 5, LI 4   **Lumbar/back** DU 3, 12, 26

Hip GB 29, 39, 30   **Thigh** BL 36, 54, GB 34

Knee Heding, Xiyan, GB 34, SP9, ST36   **Ankle** ST 41, SP5, GB40, BL 60, KD 3

Leg BL 57, 58   **Toes** SP 4, BL 65, Bafeng

General pain SI 3, BL 17, 62, SP 21, LI 4, 11, 15, TH 4, GB 30, 34, 39, ST 41

*SUPPLEMENTAL POINTS

BOIL & RED-THREAD BOIL

First a yellow or purple boil appears on the head, face or extremity.
A blister or pustula with a hard base is formed, with a tingling sensation.
Afterwards there is increased redness, swelling & pain with burning sensation, often accompanied by chills & fever.

If the boil toxicity attacks the interior:
- a red thread like line extends proximally on the boil.
- High fever
- Restlessness
- Dizziness
- Vomiting
- Impaired consciousness

T= red with yellow coat

P= rapid

DU 10,12
PC 4
LI 4
BL 40

SUPPLEMENTAL PTS
LI 1, 11, 20
GB 2, 34, 44

BREAST ABSCESS

is an acute purulent disorder found mostly during lactation after delivery. It rarely occurs during pregnancy

Redness, swelling & pain of the breast after delivery
A lump in the breast at the early stage when the abscess is unformed is accompanied by:
Swelling
Pain
Difficult lactation
Chills
Fever
Headache
Nausea
Dire thirst

GB 21
CV 17
ST 18, 36
SI 1
LV 3
SUPPLEMENTAL PTS
LI 4 - Chills & fever
GB 41 - distention & pain in breast

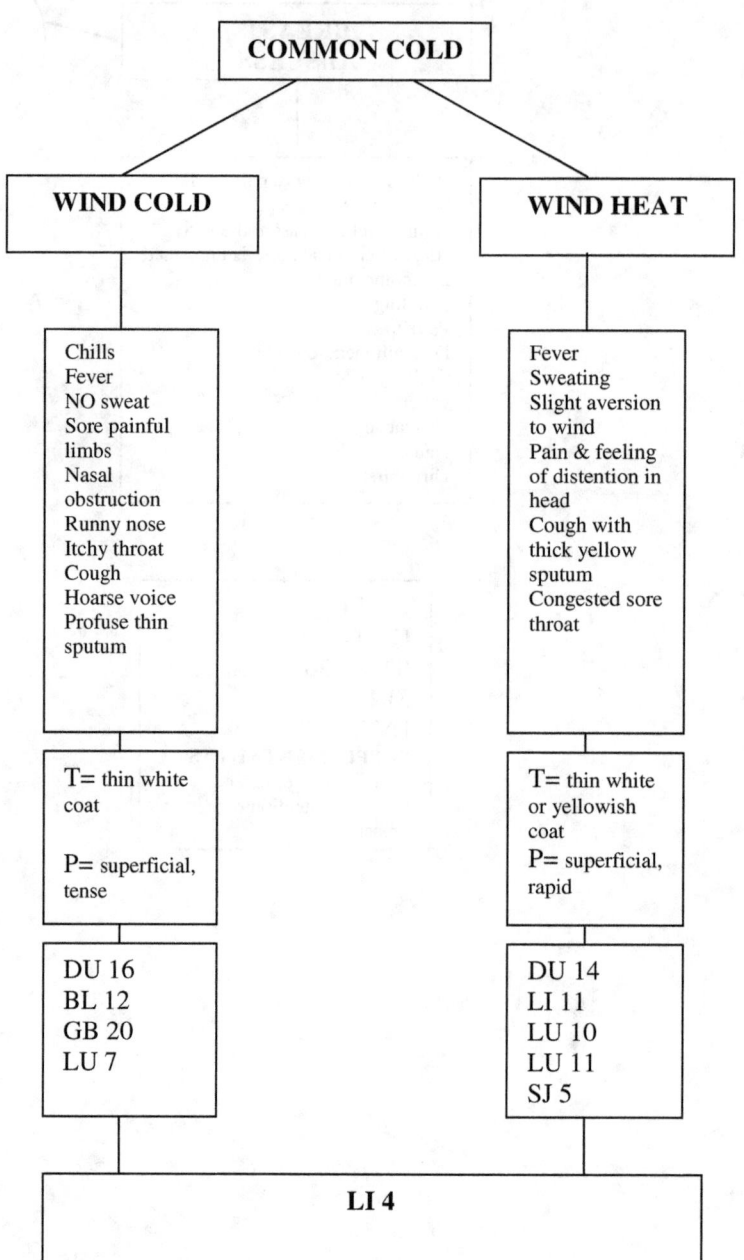

COMMON COLD

WIND COLD

Chills
Fever
NO sweat
Sore painful
limbs
Nasal
obstruction
Runny nose
Itchy throat
Cough
Hoarse voice
Profuse thin
sputum

T= thin white
coat

P= superficial,
tense

DU 16
BL 12
GB 20
LU 7

WIND HEAT

Fever
Sweating
Slight aversion
to wind
Pain & feeling
of distention in
head
Cough with
thick yellow
sputum
Congested sore
throat

T= thin white
or yellowish
coat
P= superficial,
rapid

DU 14
LI 11
LU 10
LU 11
SJ 5

LI 4

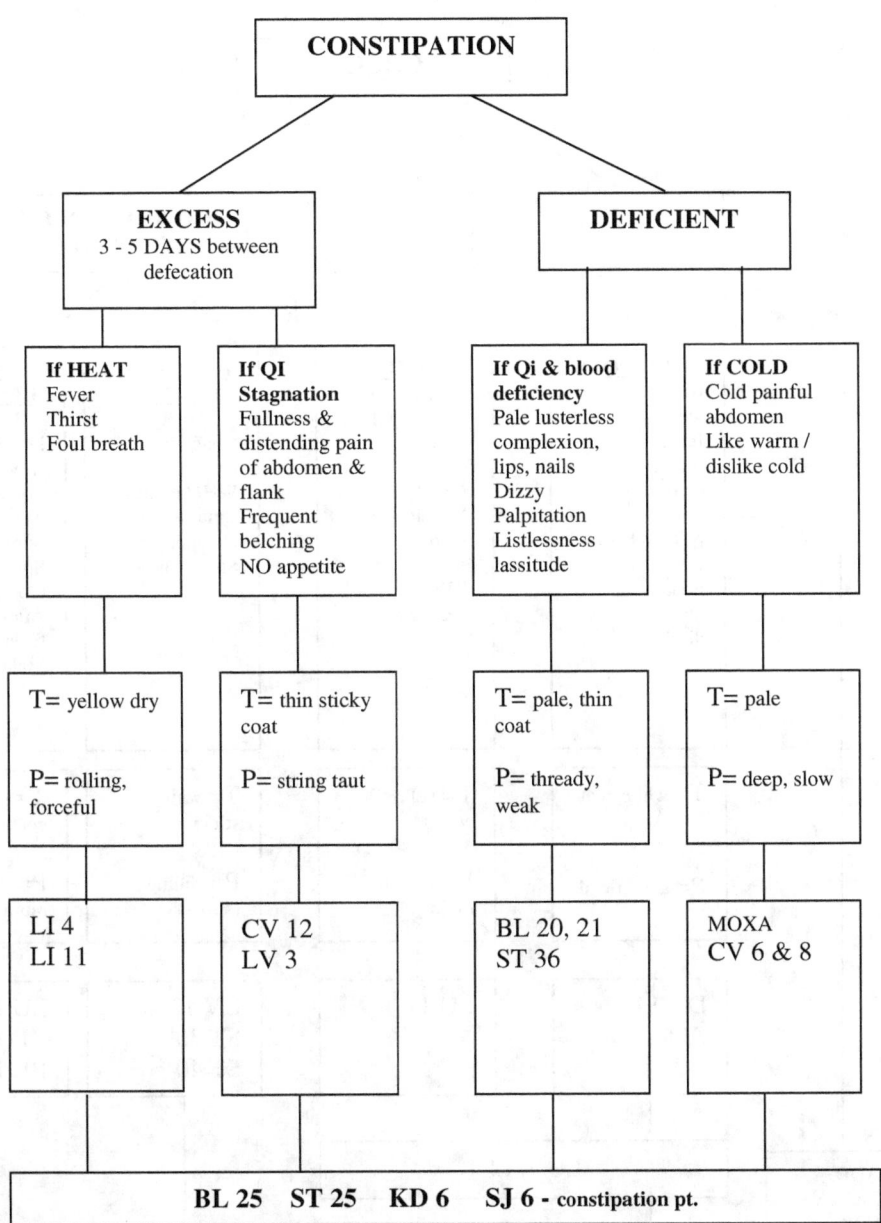

CONSTIPATION

EXCESS
3 - 5 DAYS between defecation

DEFICIENT

If HEAT
Fever
Thirst
Foul breath

If QI Stagnation
Fullness & distending pain of abdomen & flank
Frequent belching
NO appetite

If Qi & blood deficiency
Pale lusterless complexion, lips, nails
Dizzy
Palpitation
Listlessness lassitude

If COLD
Cold painful abdomen
Like warm / dislike cold

T= yellow dry

P= rolling, forceful

T= thin sticky coat

P= string taut

T= pale, thin coat

P= thready, weak

T= pale

P= deep, slow

LI 4
LI 11

CV 12
LV 3

BL 20, 21
ST 36

MOXA
CV 6 & 8

BL 25   ST 25   KD 6   SJ 6 - constipation pt.

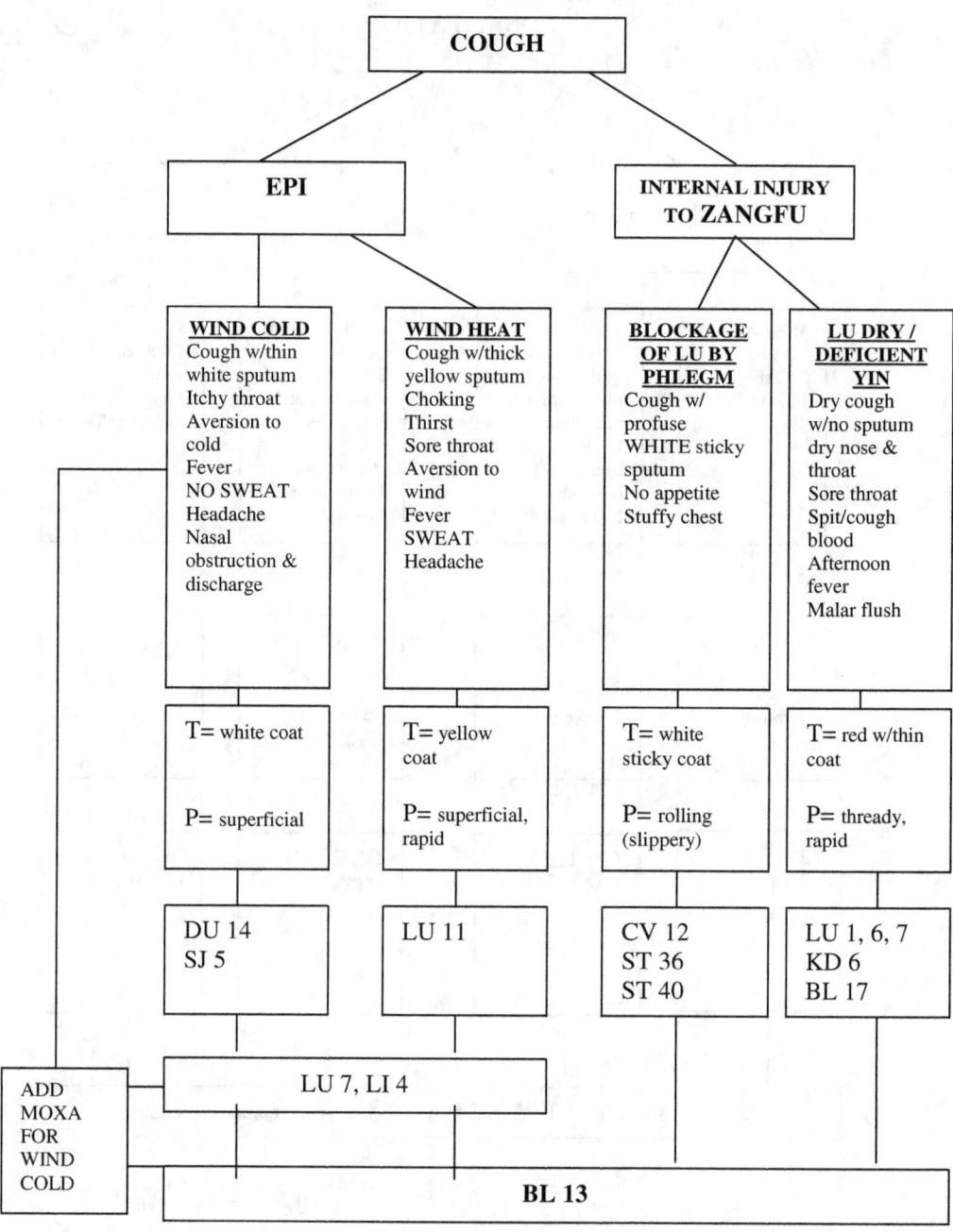

COUGH

EPI

INTERNAL INJURY TO ZANGFU

WIND COLD
Cough w/thin white sputum
Itchy throat
Aversion to cold
Fever
NO SWEAT
Headache
Nasal obstruction & discharge

WIND HEAT
Cough w/thick yellow sputum
Choking
Thirst
Sore throat
Aversion to wind
Fever
SWEAT
Headache

BLOCKAGE OF LU BY PHLEGM
Cough w/ profuse WHITE sticky sputum
No appetite
Stuffy chest

LU DRY / DEFICIENT YIN
Dry cough w/no sputum
dry nose & throat
Sore throat
Spit/cough blood
Afternoon fever
Malar flush

T= white coat

P= superficial

T= yellow coat

P= superficial, rapid

T= white sticky coat

P= rolling (slippery)

T= red w/thin coat

P= thready, rapid

DU 14
SJ 5

LU 11

CV 12
ST 36
ST 40

LU 1, 6, 7
KD 6
BL 17

ADD MOXA FOR WIND COLD

LU 7, LI 4

BL 13

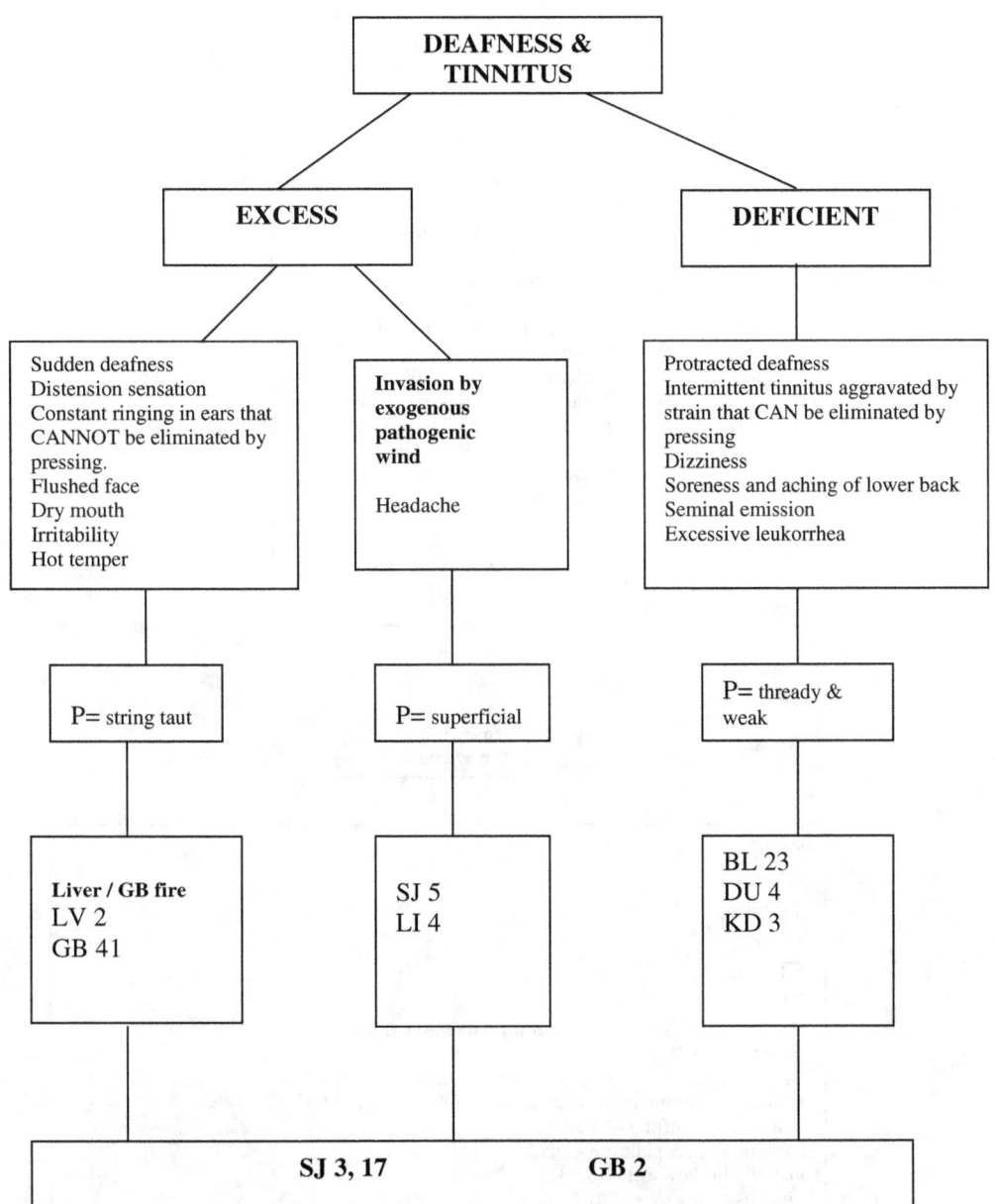

DEAFNESS & TINNITUS

EXCESS

Sudden deafness
Distension sensation
Constant ringing in ears that
CANNOT be eliminated by
pressing.
Flushed face
Dry mouth
Irritability
Hot temper

**Invasion by
exogenous
pathogenic
wind**

Headache

DEFICIENT

Protracted deafness
Intermittent tinnitus aggravated by
strain that CAN be eliminated by
pressing
Dizziness
Soreness and aching of lower back
Seminal emission
Excessive leukorrhea

P= string taut

P= superficial

P= thready &
weak

Liver / GB fire
LV 2
GB 41

SJ 5
LI 4

BL 23
DU 4
KD 3

SJ 3, 17   GB 2

DEVIATION OF THE EYE & MOUTH

Sudden onset, usually right after awakening
Incomplete closure of the eye in the affected side
Drooping of the angle of the mouth
Salivation and inability to frown, raise the eyebrow, close the eye, blow out the cheek, show the teeth or whistle, and in some cases pain in the mastoid region or headache

T= thin white coat
P= superficial tense or superficial slow

SJ 17
GB 14
Taiyang
SI 18
ST 4, 6, 7
LI 4

Supplementary points:

Headache - GB20
Difficulty in frowning & raising the eyebrow - BL2, SJ 23
Incomplete closing of the eye - BL 1, 2, GB1, Yuyao, SJ 23
Difficulty in sniffing - LI 20
Deviation of the philtrum - DU 26
Inability to show teeth - ST 3
Tinnitus & deafness - GB 2
Tenderness of the mastoid region - GB 12, SJ 5

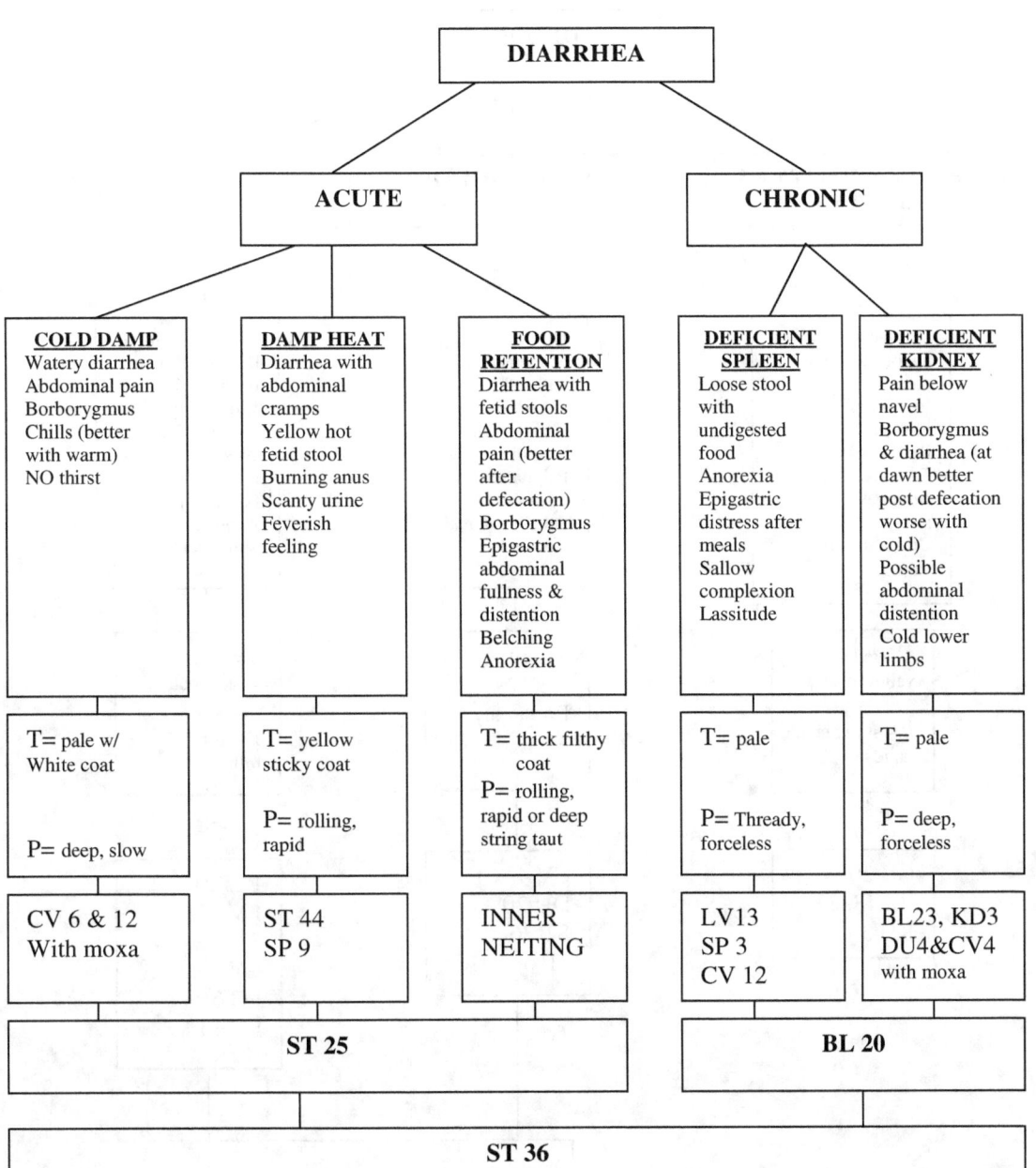

DIARRHEA

ACUTE

CHRONIC

COLD DAMP	DAMP HEAT	FOOD RETENTION	DEFICIENT SPLEEN	DEFICIENT KIDNEY
Watery diarrhea Abdominal pain Borborygmus Chills (better with warm) NO thirst	Diarrhea with abdominal cramps Yellow hot fetid stool Burning anus Scanty urine Feverish feeling	Diarrhea with fetid stools Abdominal pain (better after defecation) Borborygmus Epigastric abdominal fullness & distention Belching Anorexia	Loose stool with undigested food Anorexia Epigastric distress after meals Sallow complexion Lassitude	Pain below navel Borborygmus & diarrhea (at dawn better post defecation worse with cold) Possible abdominal distention Cold lower limbs
T= pale w/ White coat P= deep, slow	T= yellow sticky coat P= rolling, rapid	T= thick filthy coat P= rolling, rapid or deep string taut	T= pale P= Thready, forceless	T= pale P= deep, forceless
CV 6 & 12 With moxa	ST 44 SP 9	INNER NEITING	LV13 SP 3 CV 12	BL23, KD3 DU4&CV4 with moxa

ST 25 | **BL 20**

ST 36

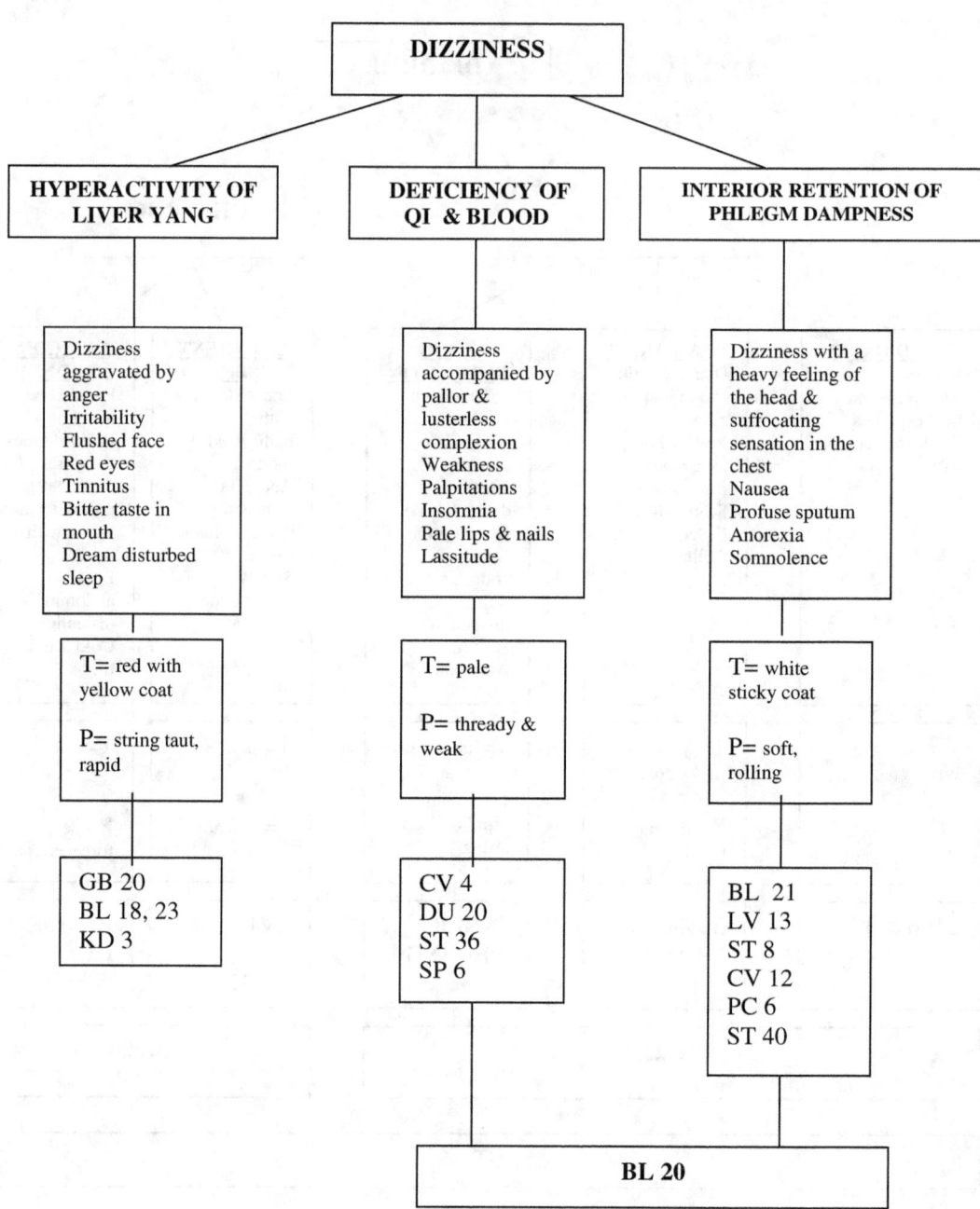

DIZZINESS

HYPERACTIVITY OF LIVER YANG

Dizziness aggravated by anger
Irritability
Flushed face
Red eyes
Tinnitus
Bitter taste in mouth
Dream disturbed sleep

T= red with yellow coat

P= string taut, rapid

GB 20
BL 18, 23
KD 3

DEFICIENCY OF QI & BLOOD

Dizziness accompanied by pallor & lusterless complexion
Weakness
Palpitations
Insomnia
Pale lips & nails
Lassitude

T= pale

P= thready & weak

CV 4
DU 20
ST 36
SP 6

INTERIOR RETENTION OF PHLEGM DAMPNESS

Dizziness with a heavy feeling of the head & suffocating sensation in the chest
Nausea
Profuse sputum
Anorexia
Somnolence

T= white sticky coat

P= soft, rolling

BL 21
LV 13
ST 8
CV 12
PC 6
ST 40

BL 20

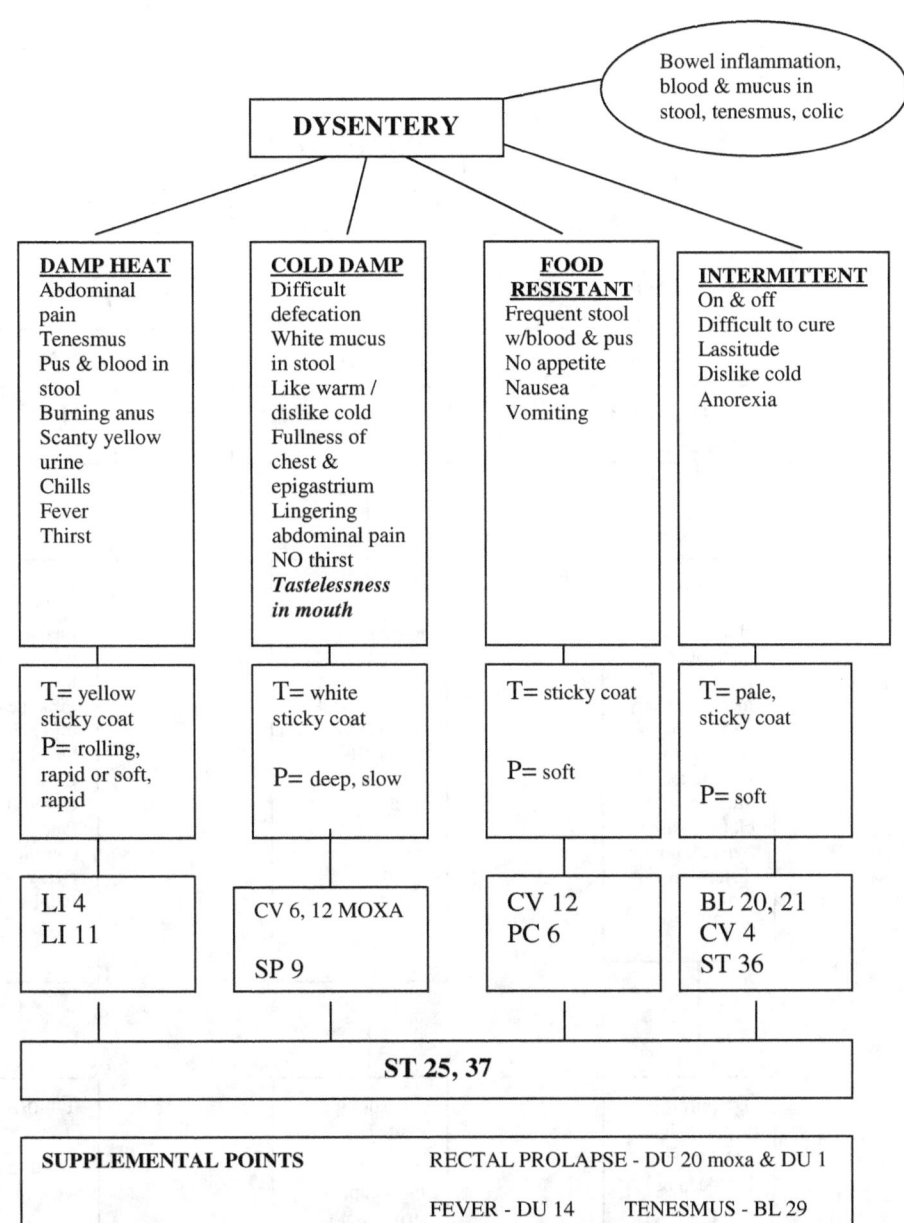

DYSENTERY

Bowel inflammation, blood & mucus in stool, tenesmus, colic

DAMP HEAT
Abdominal pain
Tenesmus
Pus & blood in stool
Burning anus
Scanty yellow urine
Chills
Fever
Thirst

COLD DAMP
Difficult defecation
White mucus in stool
Like warm / dislike cold
Fullness of chest & epigastrium
Lingering abdominal pain
NO thirst
Tastelessness in mouth

FOOD RESISTANT
Frequent stool w/blood & pus
No appetite
Nausea
Vomiting

INTERMITTENT
On & off
Difficult to cure
Lassitude
Dislike cold
Anorexia

T= yellow sticky coat
P= rolling, rapid or soft, rapid

T= white sticky coat

P= deep, slow

T= sticky coat

P= soft

T= pale, sticky coat

P= soft

LI 4
LI 11

CV 6, 12 MOXA

SP 9

CV 12
PC 6

BL 20, 21
CV 4
ST 36

ST 25, 37

SUPPLEMENTAL POINTS   RECTAL PROLAPSE - DU 20 moxa & DU 1

FEVER - DU 14   TENESMUS - BL 29

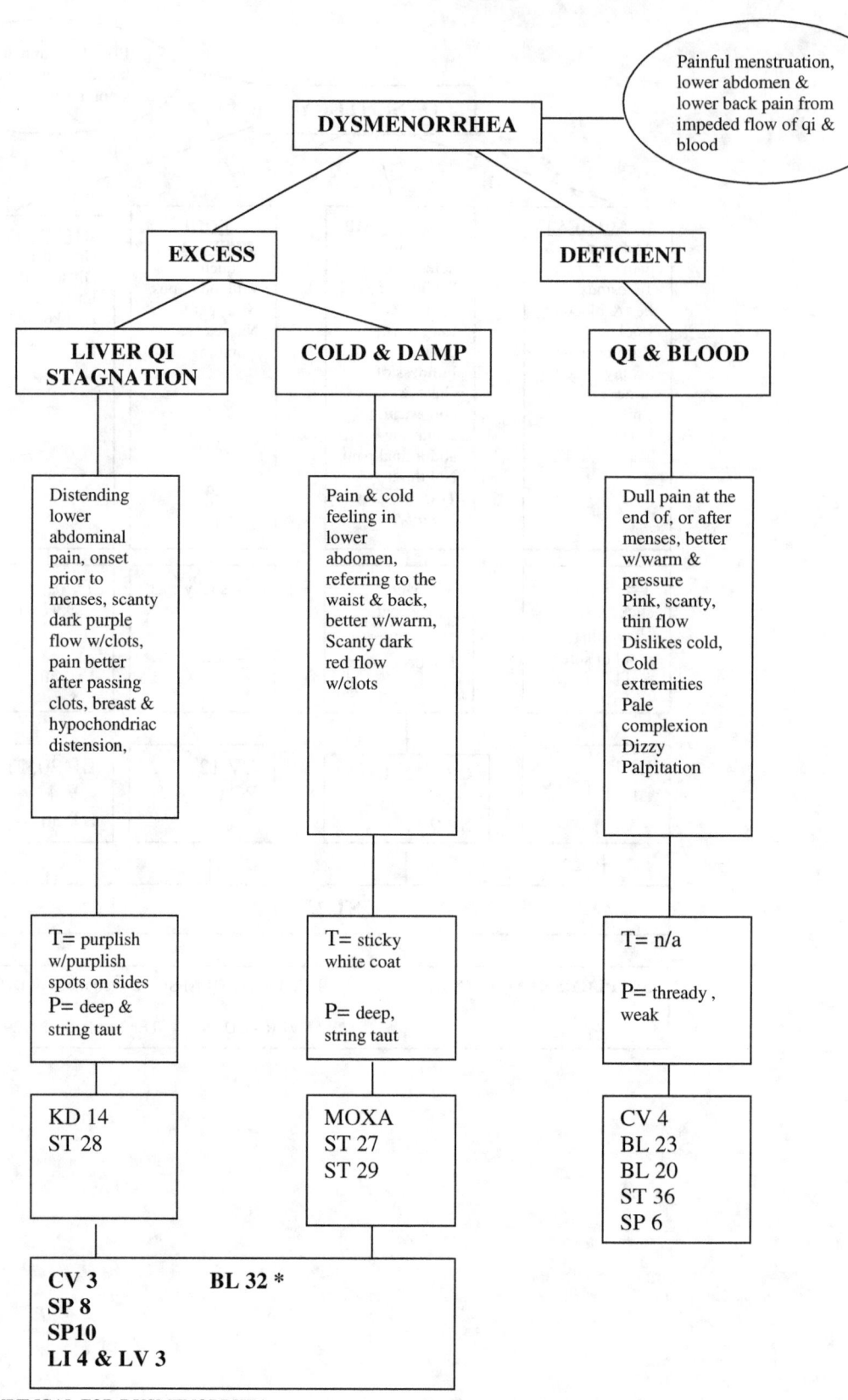

DYSMENORRHEA

Painful menstruation, lower abdomen & lower back pain from impeded flow of qi & blood

EXCESS

DEFICIENT

LIVER QI STAGNATION

COLD & DAMP

QI & BLOOD

Distending lower abdominal pain, onset prior to menses, scanty dark purple flow w/clots, pain better after passing clots, breast & hypochondriac distension,

Pain & cold feeling in lower abdomen, referring to the waist & back, better w/warm, Scanty dark red flow w/clots

Dull pain at the end of, or after menses, better w/warm & pressure Pink, scanty, thin flow Dislikes cold, Cold extremities Pale complexion Dizzy Palpitation

T= purplish w/purplish spots on sides
P= deep & string taut

T= sticky white coat

P= deep, string taut

T= n/a

P= thready , weak

KD 14
ST 28

MOXA
ST 27
ST 29

CV 4
BL 23
BL 20
ST 36
SP 6

CV 3   BL 32 *
SP 8
SP10
LI 4 & LV 3

* EMPIRICAL FOR DYSMENORRHEA

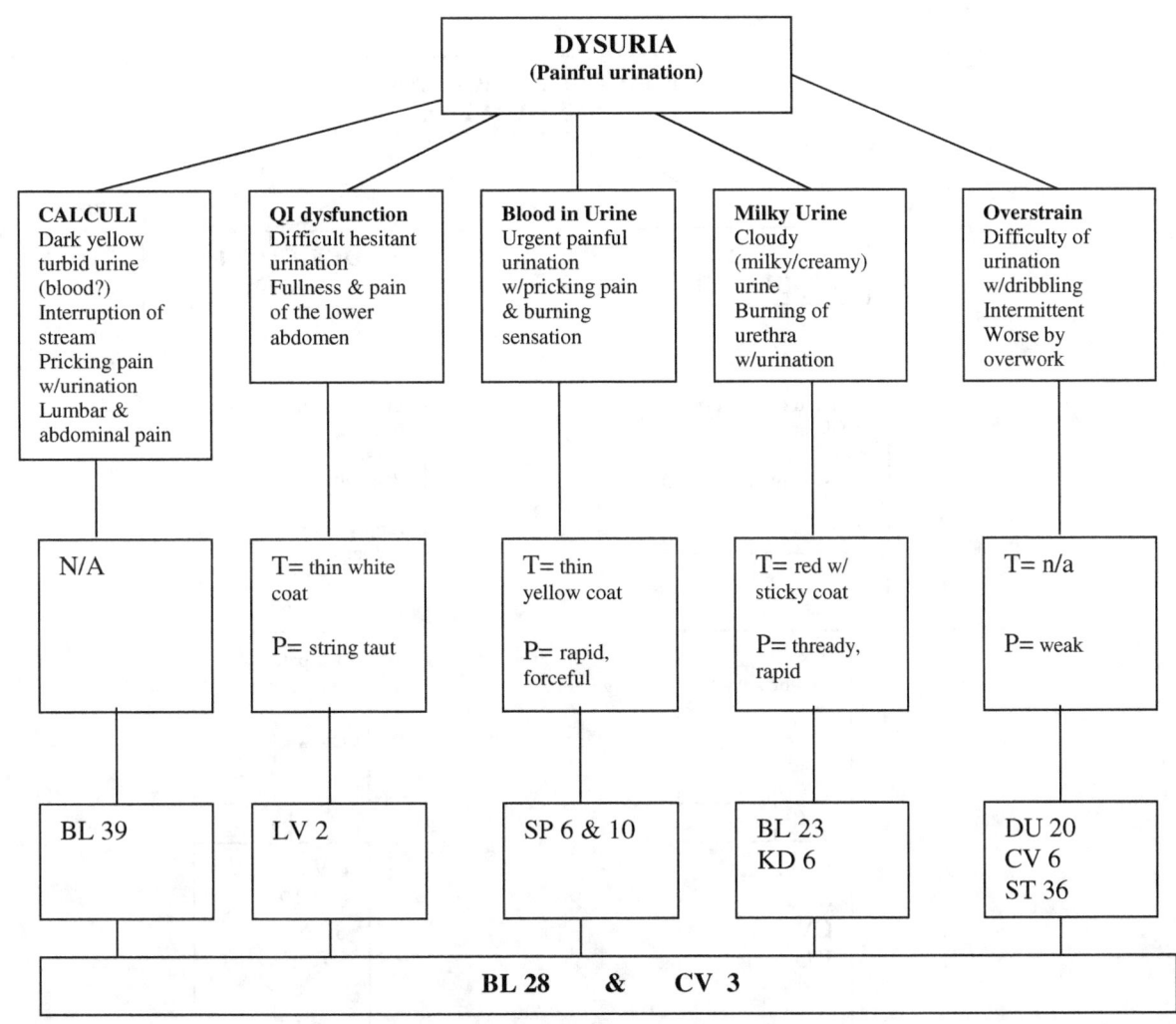

DYSURIA
(Painful urination)

CALCULI	QI dysfunction	Blood in Urine	Milky Urine	Overstrain
Dark yellow turbid urine (blood?) Interruption of stream Pricking pain w/urination Lumbar & abdominal pain	Difficult hesitant urination Fullness & pain of the lower abdomen	Urgent painful urination w/pricking pain & burning sensation	Cloudy (milky/creamy) urine Burning of urethra w/urination	Difficulty of urination w/dribbling Intermittent Worse by overwork

| N/A | T= thin white coat P= string taut | T= thin yellow coat P= rapid, forceful | T= red w/ sticky coat P= thready, rapid | T= n/a P= weak |

| BL 39 | LV 2 | SP 6 & 10 | BL 23 KD 6 | DU 20 CV 6 ST 36 |

BL 28 & CV 3

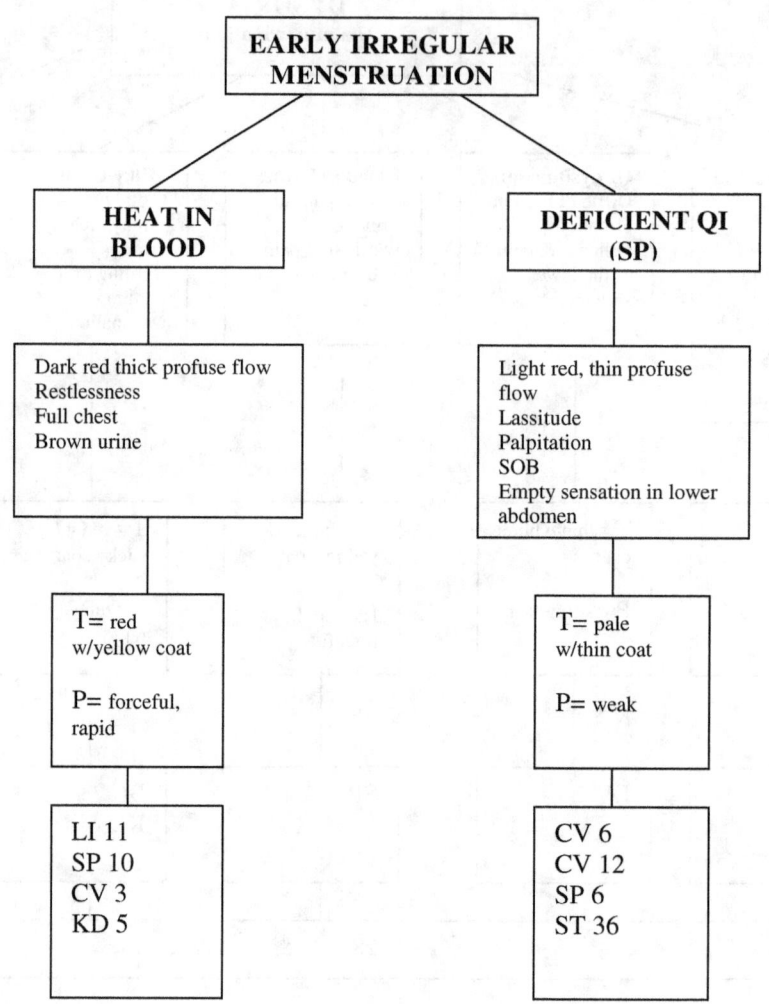

EARLY IRREGULAR MENSTRUATION

HEAT IN BLOOD

Dark red thick profuse flow
Restlessness
Full chest
Brown urine

T= red
w/yellow coat

P= forceful,
rapid

LI 11
SP 10
CV 3
KD 5

DEFICIENT QI (SP)

Light red, thin profuse flow
Lassitude
Palpitation
SOB
Empty sensation in lower abdomen

T= pale
w/thin coat

P= weak

CV 6
CV 12
SP 6
ST 36

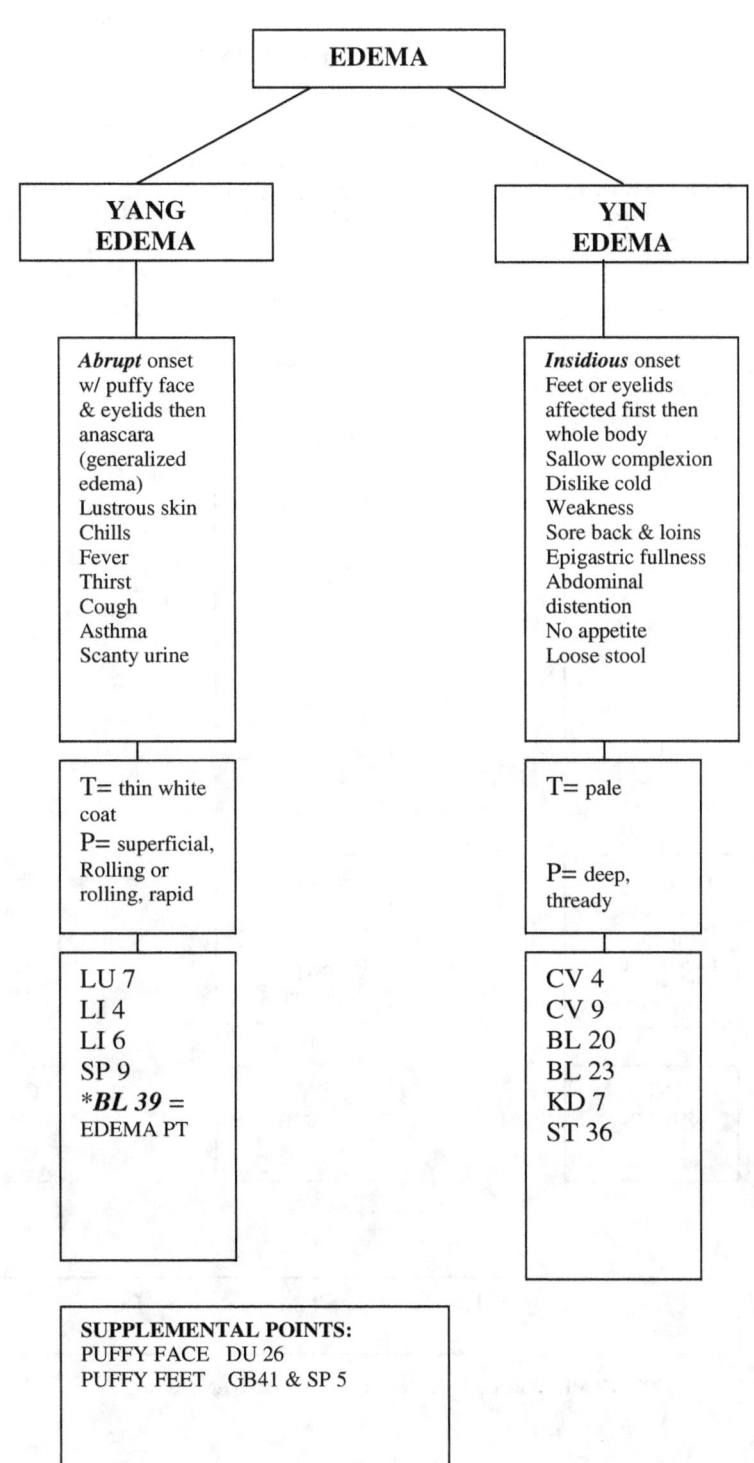

EDEMA

YANG EDEMA

YIN EDEMA

Abrupt onset
w/ puffy face
& eyelids then
anascara
(generalized
edema)
Lustrous skin
Chills
Fever
Thirst
Cough
Asthma
Scanty urine

Insidious onset
Feet or eyelids
affected first then
whole body
Sallow complexion
Dislike cold
Weakness
Sore back & loins
Epigastric fullness
Abdominal
distention
No appetite
Loose stool

T= thin white
coat
P= superficial,
Rolling or
rolling, rapid

T= pale

P= deep,
thready

LU 7
LI 4
LI 6
SP 9
BL 39 =
EDEMA PT

CV 4
CV 9
BL 20
BL 23
KD 7
ST 36

SUPPLEMENTAL POINTS:
PUFFY FACE   DU 26
PUFFY FEET   GB41 & SP 5

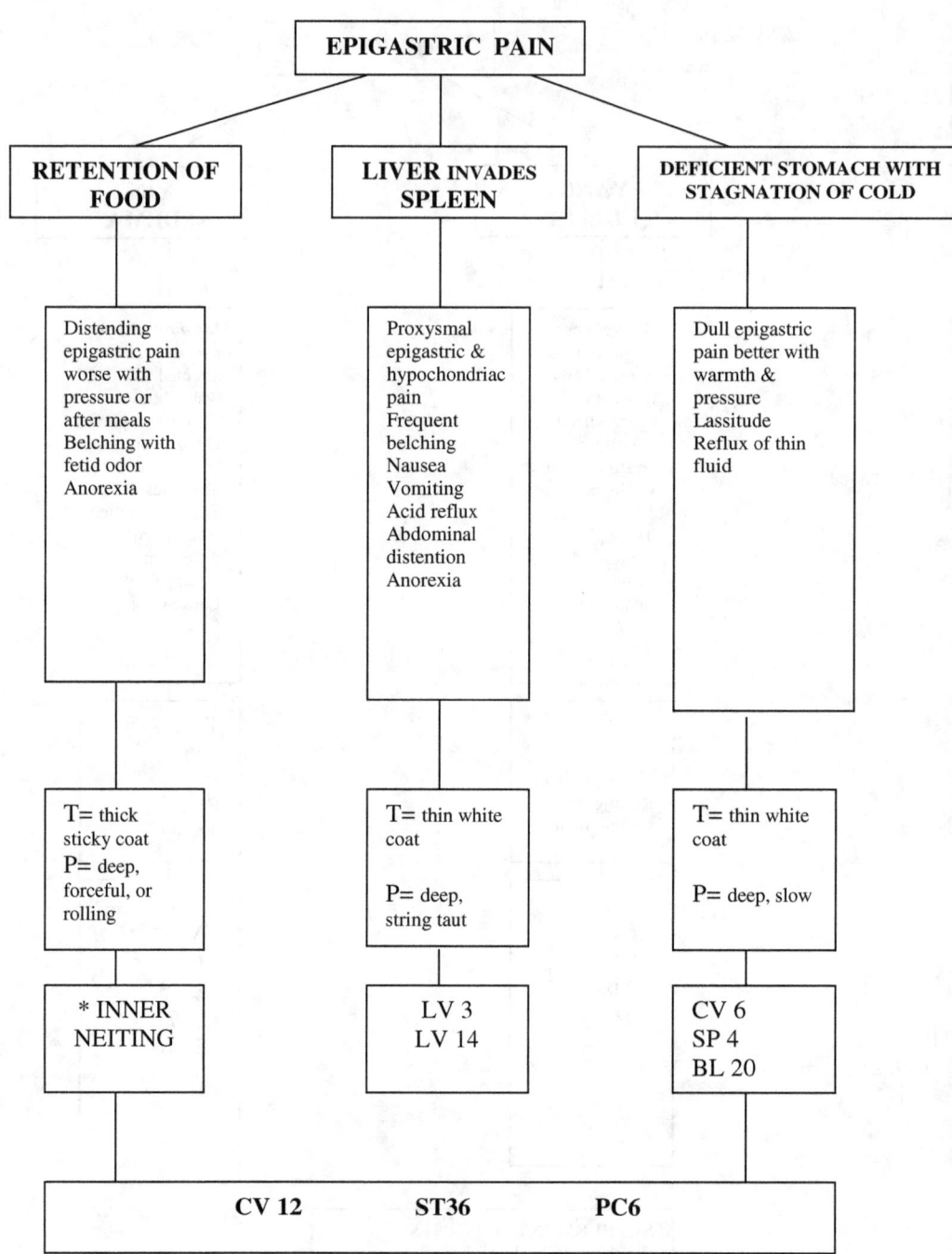

EPIGASTRIC PAIN

RETENTION OF FOOD

LIVER INVADES SPLEEN

DEFICIENT STOMACH WITH STAGNATION OF COLD

Distending epigastric pain worse with pressure or after meals
Belching with fetid odor
Anorexia

Proxysmal epigastric & hypochondriac pain
Frequent belching
Nausea
Vomiting
Acid reflux
Abdominal distention
Anorexia

Dull epigastric pain better with warmth & pressure
Lassitude
Reflux of thin fluid

T= thick sticky coat
P= deep, forceful, or rolling

T= thin white coat

P= deep, string taut

T= thin white coat

P= deep, slow

* INNER NEITING

LV 3
LV 14

CV 6
SP 4
BL 20

| CV 12 | ST36 | PC6 |

*EXTRA EMPIRICAL POINT FOR FOOD RETENTION

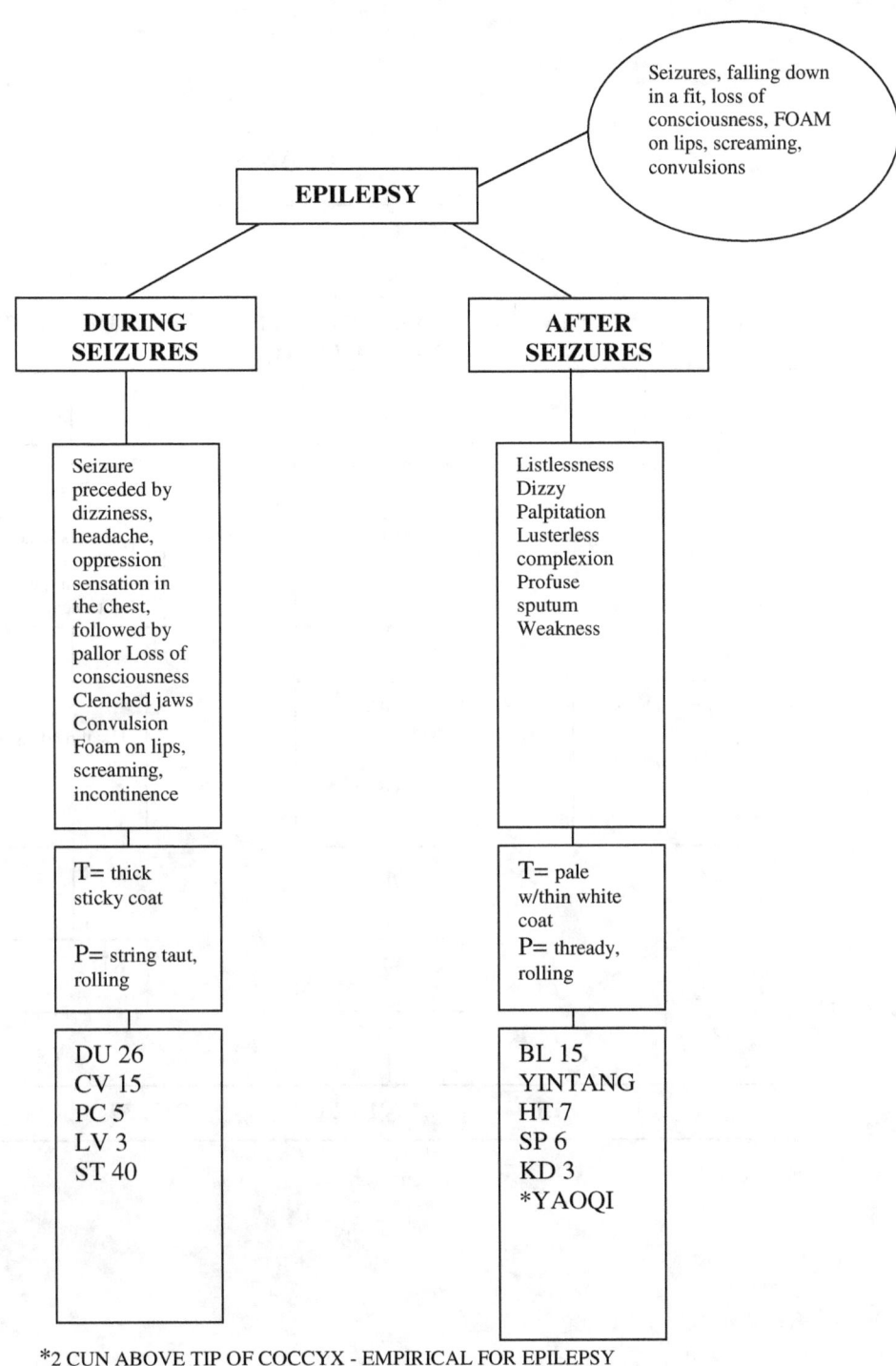

EPILEPSY

Seizures, falling down in a fit, loss of consciousness, FOAM on lips, screaming, convulsions

DURING SEIZURES

AFTER SEIZURES

Seizure preceded by dizziness, headache, oppression sensation in the chest, followed by pallor Loss of consciousness Clenched jaws Convulsion Foam on lips, screaming, incontinence

Listlessness
Dizzy
Palpitation
Lusterless complexion
Profuse sputum
Weakness

T= thick sticky coat

P= string taut, rolling

T= pale w/thin white coat
P= thready, rolling

DU 26
CV 15
PC 5
LV 3
ST 40

BL 15
YINTANG
HT 7
SP 6
KD 3
*YAOQI

*2 CUN ABOVE TIP OF COCCYX - EMPIRICAL FOR EPILEPSY

SUPPLEMENTAL POINTS:
Daytime seizures BL 62
Night seizures   KD 6
Phlegm stagnation CV 12, ST 40
Severe deficiency of Qi & Blood
                   CV4, ST 36

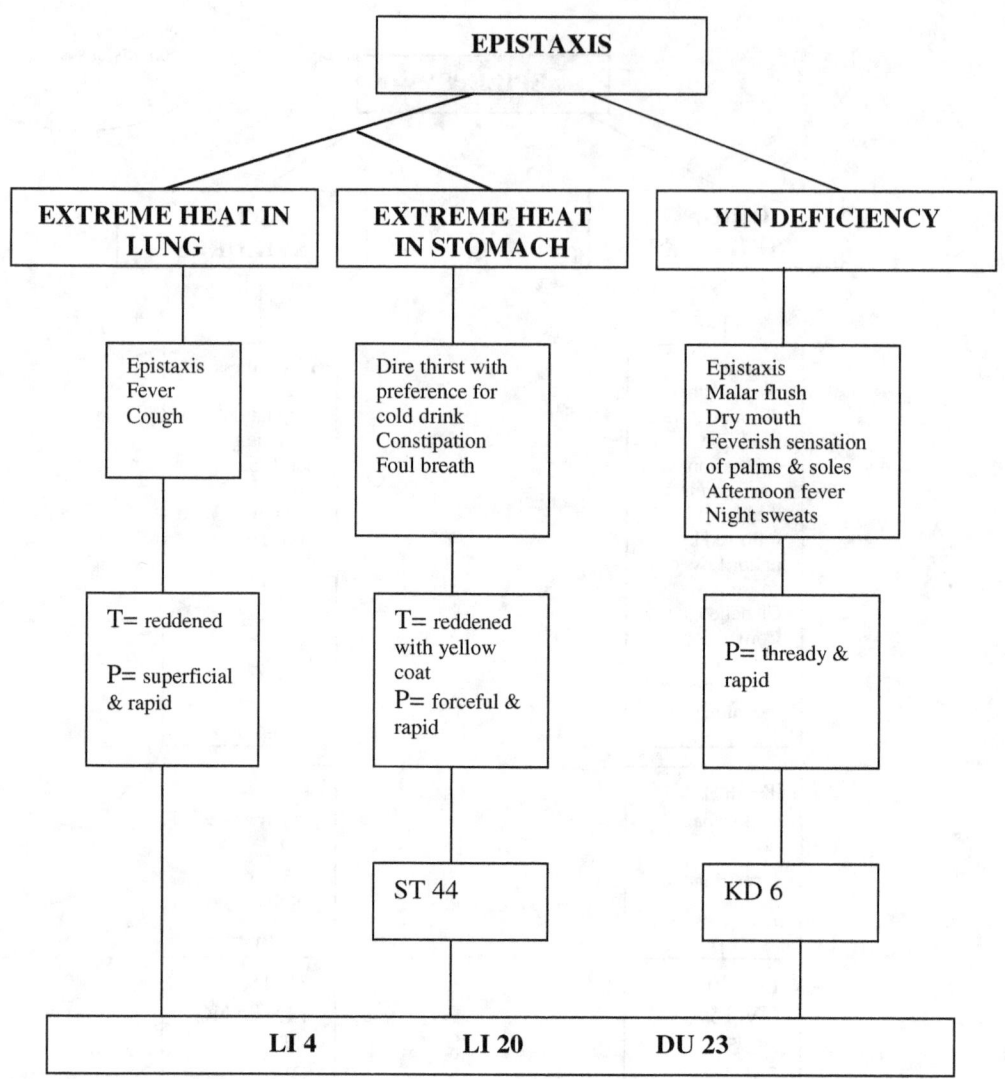

EPISTAXIS

| EXTREME HEAT IN LUNG | EXTREME HEAT IN STOMACH | YIN DEFICIENCY |

Epistaxis
Fever
Cough

Dire thirst with
preference for
cold drink
Constipation
Foul breath

Epistaxis
Malar flush
Dry mouth
Feverish sensation
of palms & soles
Afternoon fever
Night sweats

T= reddened

P= superficial
& rapid

T= reddened
with yellow
coat
P= forceful &
rapid

P= thready &
rapid

ST 44

KD 6

LI 4   LI 20   DU 23

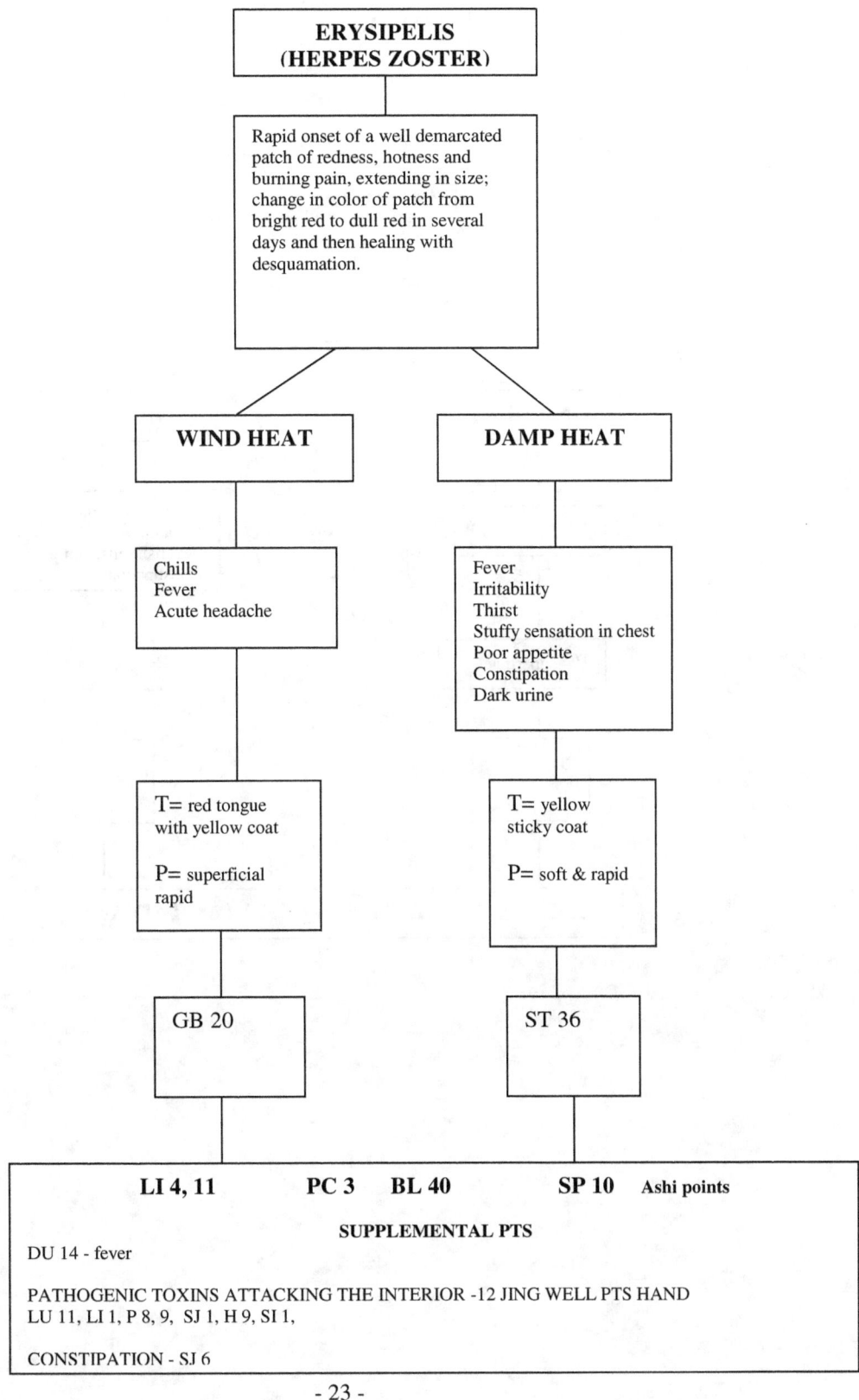

ERYSIPELIS (HERPES ZOSTER)

Rapid onset of a well demarcated patch of redness, hotness and burning pain, extending in size; change in color of patch from bright red to dull red in several days and then healing with desquamation.

WIND HEAT

Chills
Fever
Acute headache

T= red tongue
with yellow coat

P= superficial
rapid

GB 20

DAMP HEAT

Fever
Irritability
Thirst
Stuffy sensation in chest
Poor appetite
Constipation
Dark urine

T= yellow
sticky coat

P= soft & rapid

ST 36

LI 4, 11   **PC 3**   **BL 40**   **SP 10**   **Ashi points**

SUPPLEMENTAL PTS

DU 14 - fever

PATHOGENIC TOXINS ATTACKING THE INTERIOR -12 JING WELL PTS HAND
LU 11, LI 1, P 8, 9, SJ 1, H 9, SI 1,

CONSTIPATION - SJ 6

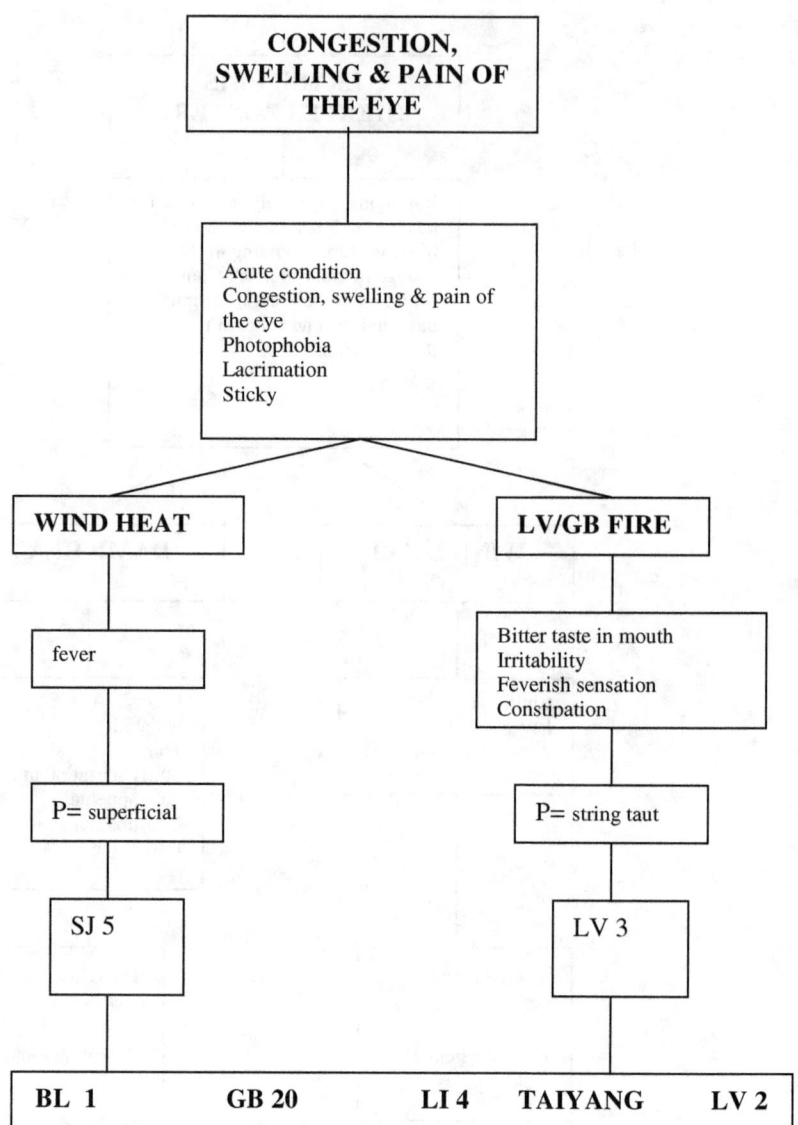

CONGESTION, SWELLING & PAIN OF THE EYE

Acute condition
Congestion, swelling & pain of the eye
Photophobia
Lacrimation
Sticky

WIND HEAT

fever

P= superficial

SJ 5

LV/GB FIRE

Bitter taste in mouth
Irritability
Feverish sensation
Constipation

P= string taut

LV 3

BL 1   GB 20   LI 4   TAIYANG   LV 2

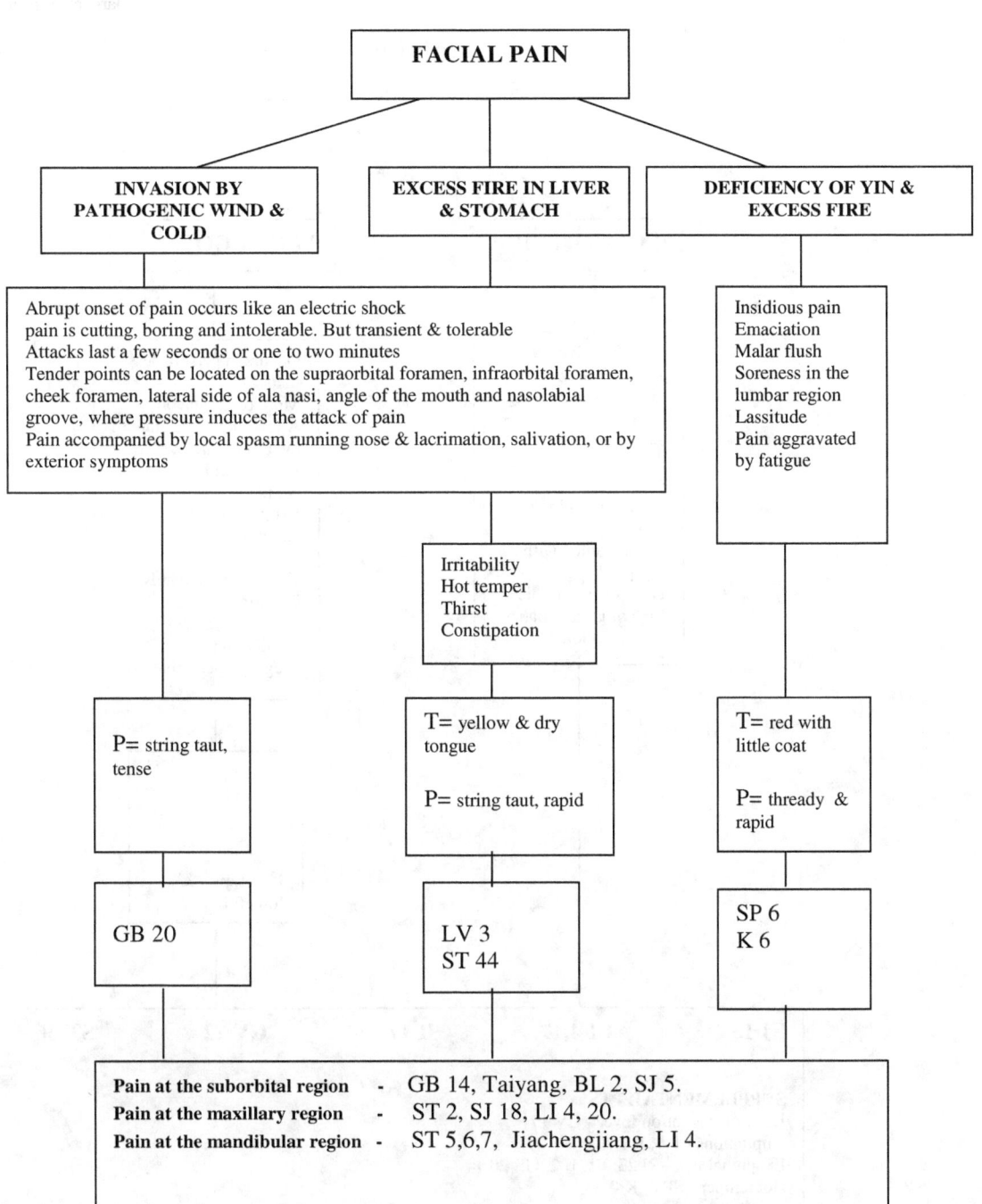

FACIAL PAIN

INVASION BY PATHOGENIC WIND & COLD

EXCESS FIRE IN LIVER & STOMACH

DEFICIENCY OF YIN & EXCESS FIRE

Abrupt onset of pain occurs like an electric shock
pain is cutting, boring and intolerable. But transient & tolerable
Attacks last a few seconds or one to two minutes
Tender points can be located on the supraorbital foramen, infraorbital foramen,
cheek foramen, lateral side of ala nasi, angle of the mouth and nasolabial
groove, where pressure induces the attack of pain
Pain accompanied by local spasm running nose & lacrimation, salivation, or by
exterior symptoms

Insidious pain
Emaciation
Malar flush
Soreness in the
lumbar region
Lassitude
Pain aggravated
by fatigue

Irritability
Hot temper
Thirst
Constipation

P= string taut,
tense

T= yellow & dry
tongue

P= string taut, rapid

T= red with
little coat

P= thready &
rapid

GB 20

LV 3
ST 44

SP 6
K 6

Pain at the suborbital region	-	GB 14, Taiyang, BL 2, SJ 5.
Pain at the maxillary region	-	ST 2, SJ 18, LI 4, 20.
Pain at the mandibular region	-	ST 5,6,7, Jiachengjiang, LI 4.

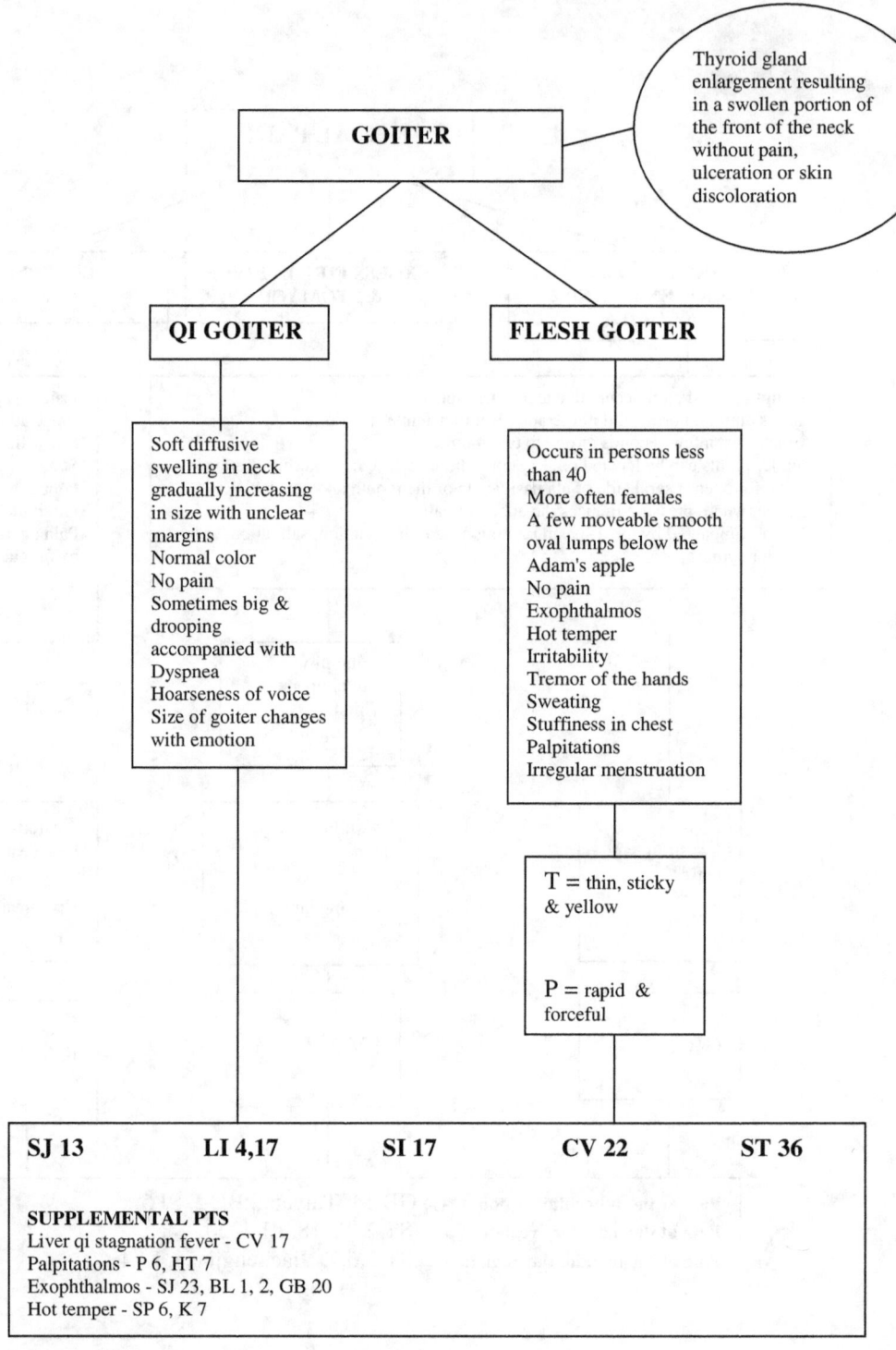

GOITER

Thyroid gland enlargement resulting in a swollen portion of the front of the neck without pain, ulceration or skin discoloration

QI GOITER

Soft diffusive swelling in neck gradually increasing in size with unclear margins
Normal color
No pain
Sometimes big & drooping accompanied with Dyspnea
Hoarseness of voice
Size of goiter changes with emotion

FLESH GOITER

Occurs in persons less than 40
More often females
A few moveable smooth oval lumps below the Adam's apple
No pain
Exophthalmos
Hot temper
Irritability
Tremor of the hands
Sweating
Stuffiness in chest
Palpitations
Irregular menstruation

T = thin, sticky & yellow

P = rapid & forceful

| SJ 13 | LI 4,17 | SI 17 | CV 22 | ST 36 |

SUPPLEMENTAL PTS
Liver qi stagnation fever - CV 17
Palpitations - P 6, HT 7
Exophthalmos - SJ 23, BL 1, 2, GB 20
Hot temper - SP 6, K 7

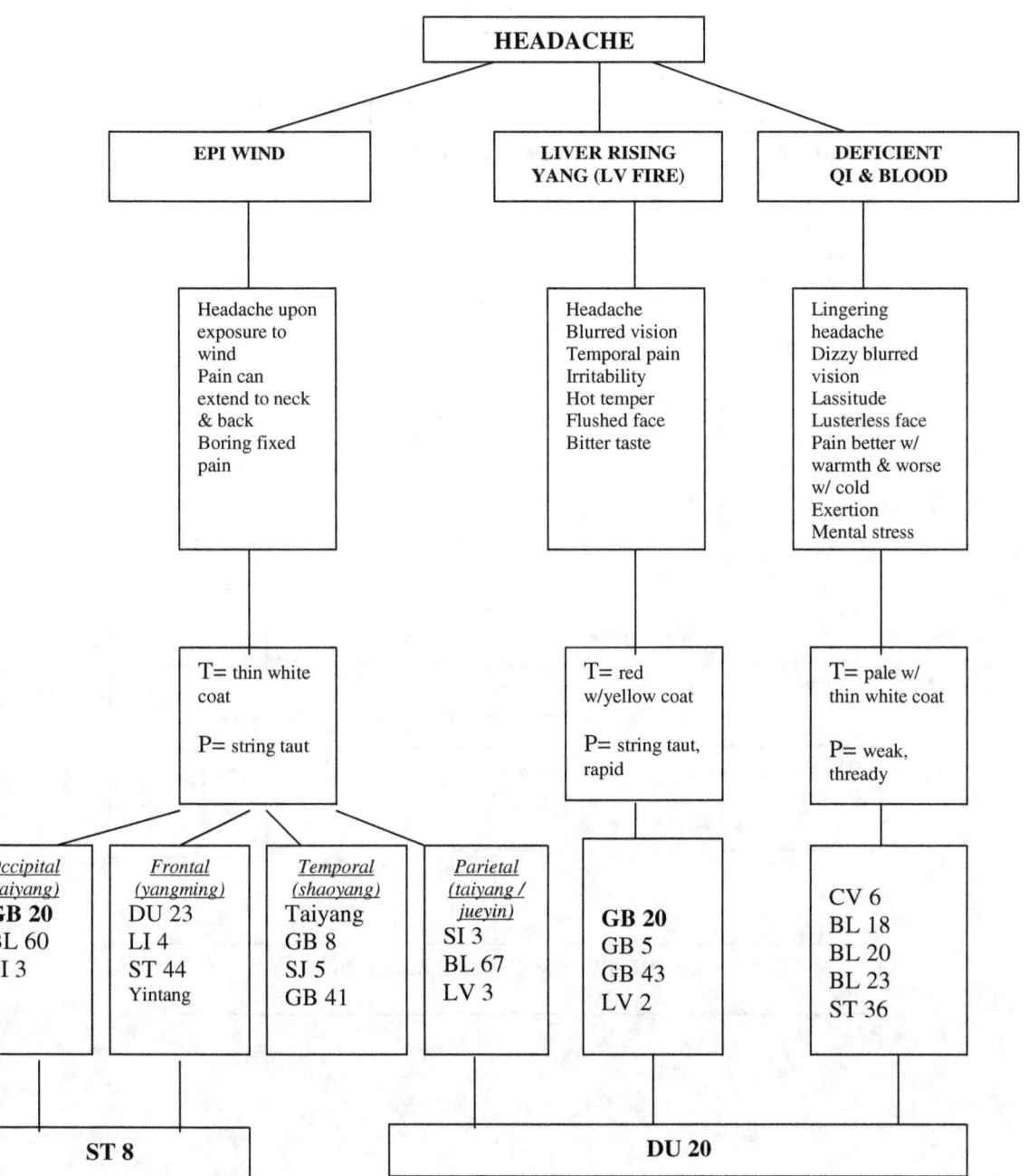

HEADACHE

EPI WIND

Headache upon
exposure to
wind
Pain can
extend to neck
& back
Boring fixed
pain

T= thin white
coat

P= string taut

*Occipital
(taiyang)*
GB 20
BL 60
SI 3

*Frontal
(yangming)*
DU 23
LI 4
ST 44
Yintang

*Temporal
(shaoyang)*
Taiyang
GB 8
SJ 5
GB 41

*Parietal
(taiyang /
jueyin)*
SI 3
BL 67
LV 3

ST 8

**LIVER RISING
YANG (LV FIRE)**

Headache
Blurred vision
Temporal pain
Irritability
Hot temper
Flushed face
Bitter taste

T= red
w/yellow coat

P= string taut,
rapid

GB 20
GB 5
GB 43
LV 2

DU 20

**DEFICIENT
QI & BLOOD**

Lingering
headache
Dizzy blurred
vision
Lassitude
Lusterless face
Pain better w/
warmth & worse
w/ cold
Exertion
Mental stress

T= pale w/
thin white coat

P= weak,
thready

CV 6
BL 18
BL 20
BL 23
ST 36

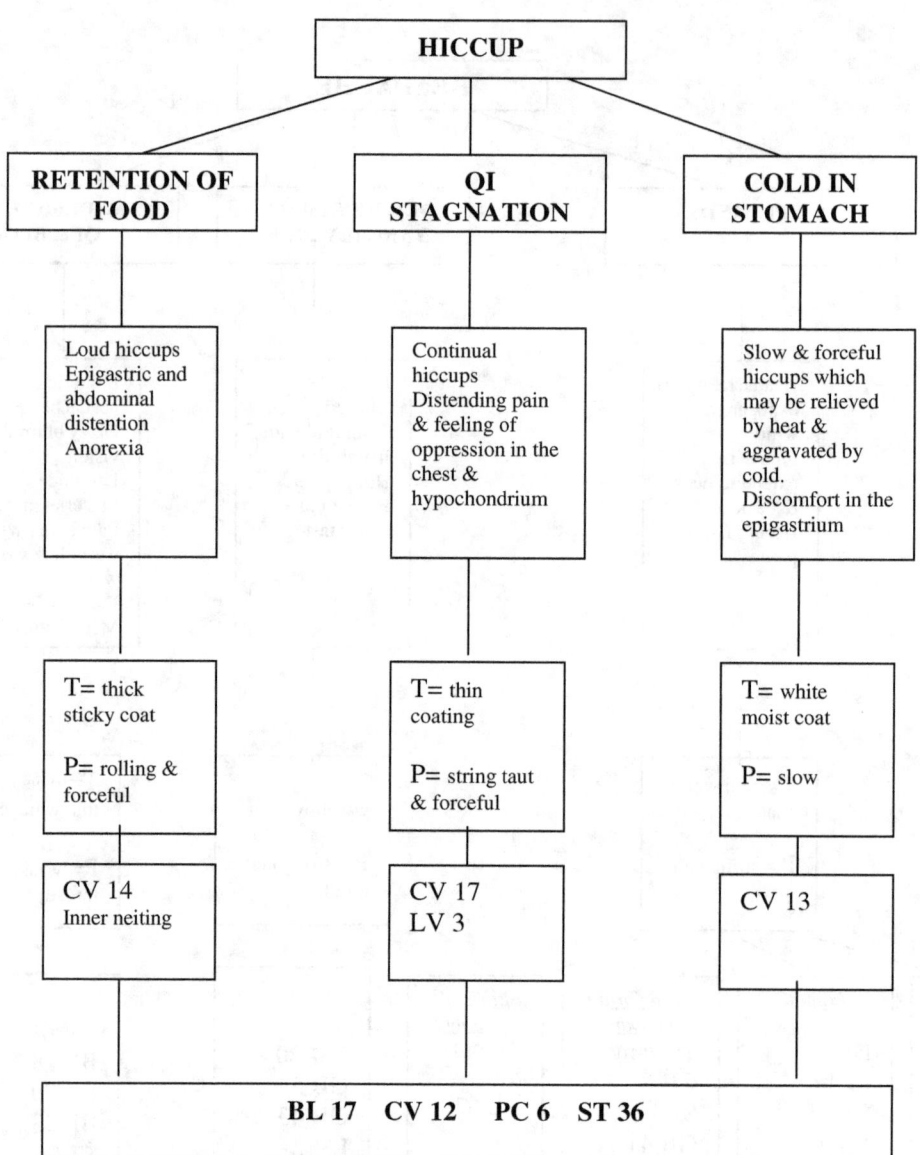

HICCUP

RETENTION OF FOOD

QI STAGNATION

COLD IN STOMACH

Loud hiccups
Epigastric and
abdominal
distention
Anorexia

Continual
hiccups
Distending pain
& feeling of
oppression in the
chest &
hypochondrium

Slow & forceful
hiccups which
may be relieved
by heat &
aggravated by
cold.
Discomfort in the
epigastrium

T= thick
sticky coat

P= rolling &
forceful

T= thin
coating

P= string taut
& forceful

T= white
moist coat

P= slow

CV 14
Inner neiting

CV 17
LV 3

CV 13

BL 17   CV 12   PC 6   ST 36

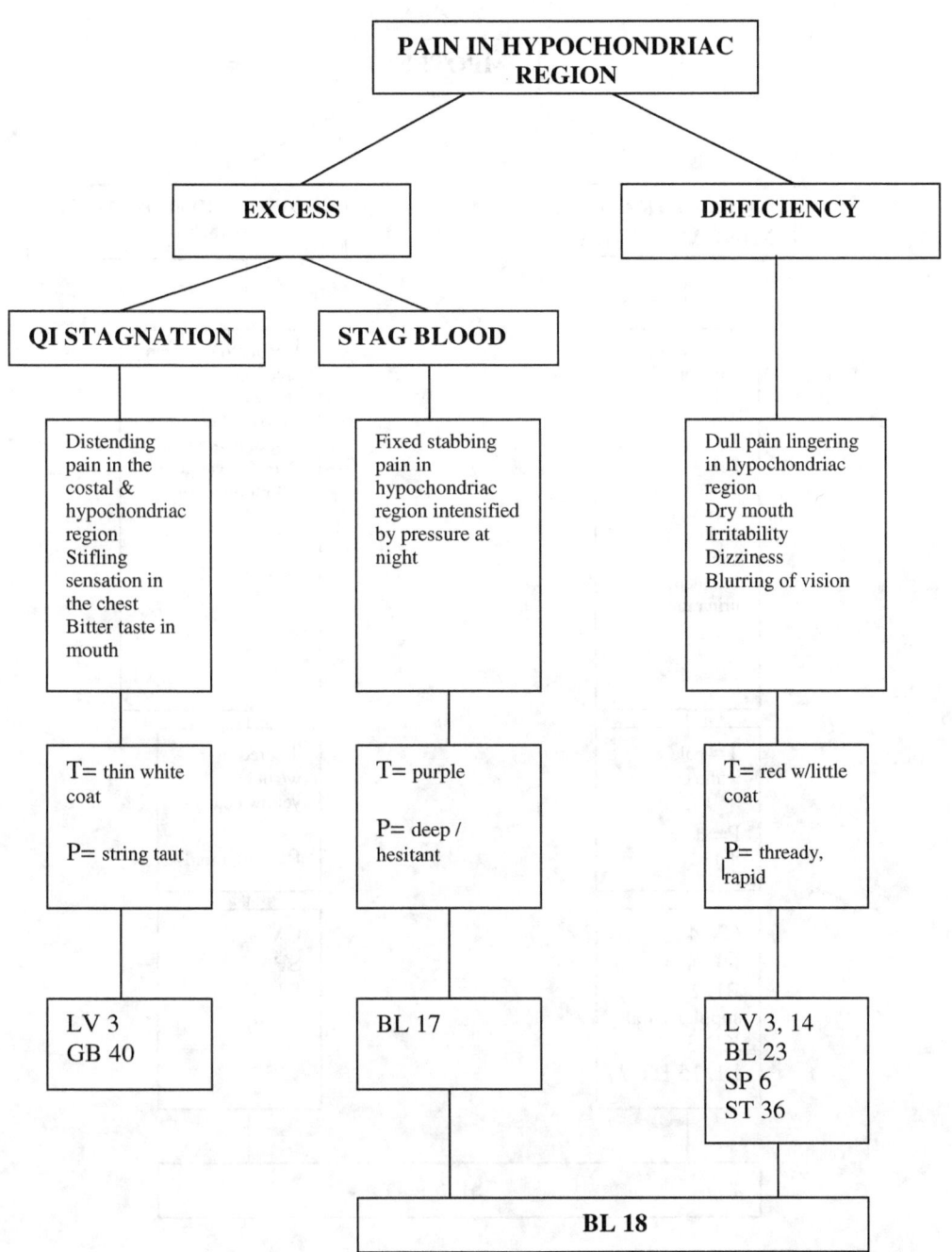

PAIN IN HYPOCHONDRIAC REGION

EXCESS

DEFICIENCY

QI STAGNATION

STAG BLOOD

Distending pain in the costal & hypochondriac region
Stifling sensation in the chest
Bitter taste in mouth

Fixed stabbing pain in hypochondriac region intensified by pressure at night

Dull pain lingering in hypochondriac region
Dry mouth
Irritability
Dizziness
Blurring of vision

T= thin white coat

P= string taut

T= purple

P= deep / hesitant

T= red w/little coat

P= thready, rapid

LV 3
GB 40

BL 17

LV 3, 14
BL 23
SP 6
ST 36

BL 18

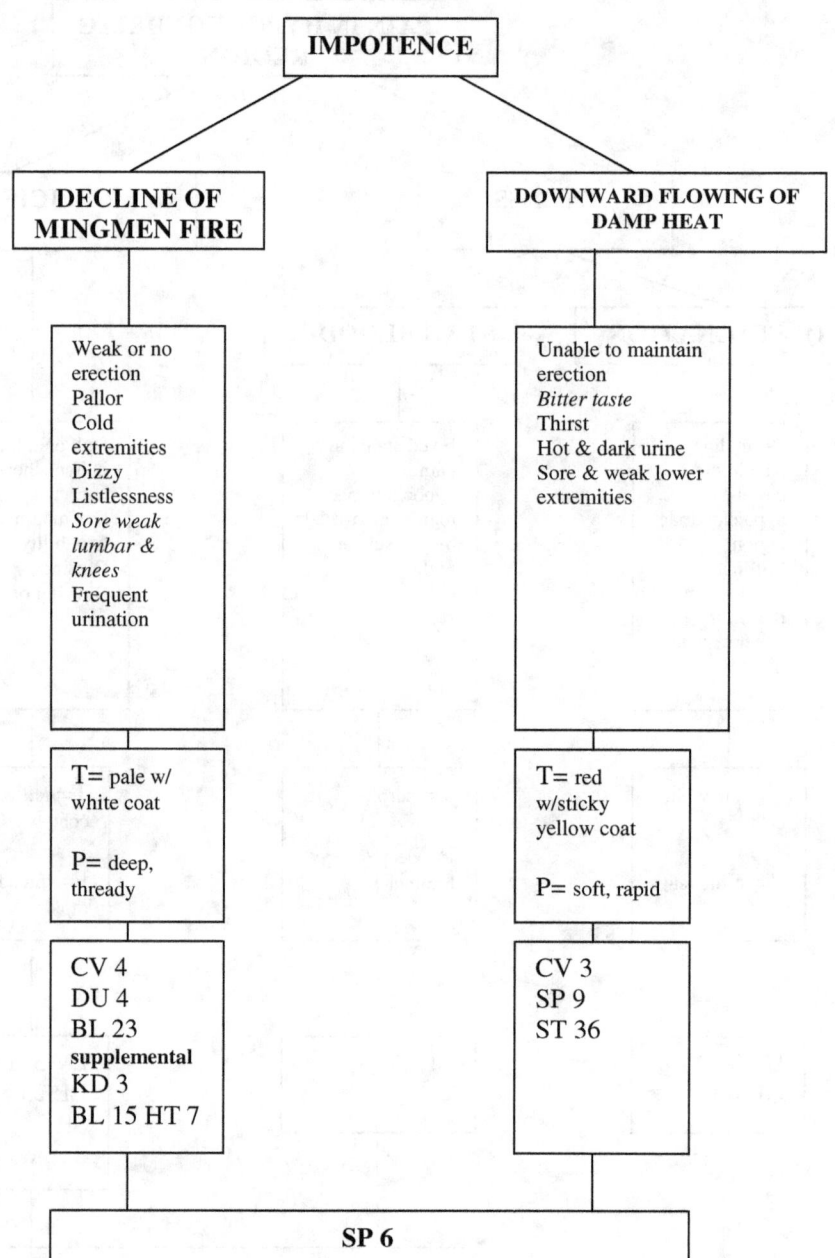

IMPOTENCE

DECLINE OF MINGMEN FIRE

Weak or no
erection
Pallor
Cold
extremities
Dizzy
Listlessness
*Sore weak
lumbar &
knees*
Frequent
urination

T= pale w/
white coat

P= deep,
thready

CV 4
DU 4
BL 23
supplemental
KD 3
BL 15 HT 7

DOWNWARD FLOWING OF DAMP HEAT

Unable to maintain
erection
Bitter taste
Thirst
Hot & dark urine
Sore & weak lower
extremities

T= red
w/sticky
yellow coat

P= soft, rapid

CV 3
SP 9
ST 36

SP 6

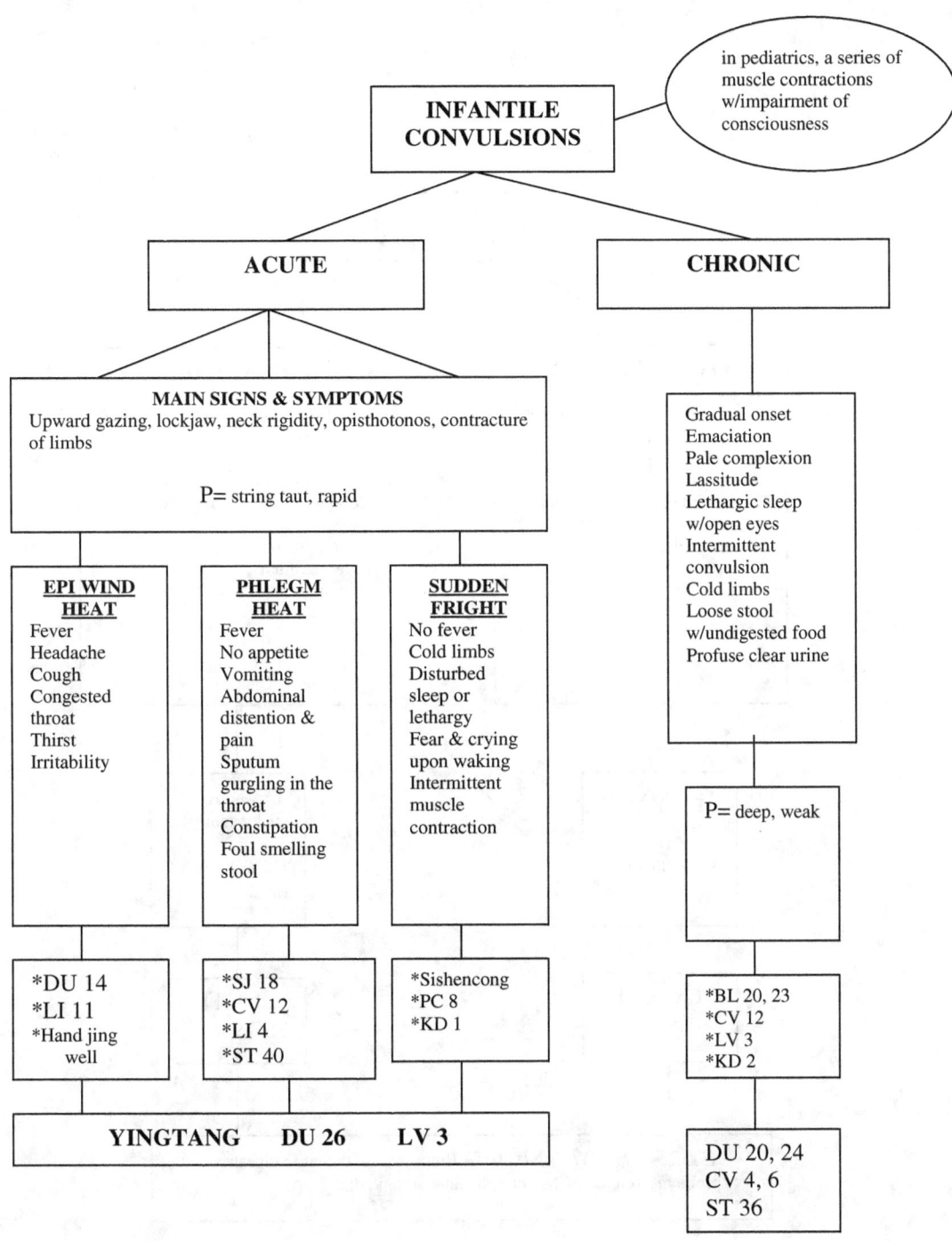

INFANTILE CONVULSIONS

in pediatrics, a series of muscle contractions w/impairment of consciousness

ACUTE

CHRONIC

MAIN SIGNS & SYMPTOMS
Upward gazing, lockjaw, neck rigidity, opisthotonos, contracture of limbs

P= string taut, rapid

EPI WIND HEAT
Fever
Headache
Cough
Congested throat
Thirst
Irritability

PHLEGM HEAT
Fever
No appetite
Vomiting
Abdominal distention & pain
Sputum gurgling in the throat
Constipation
Foul smelling stool

SUDDEN FRIGHT
No fever
Cold limbs
Disturbed sleep or lethargy
Fear & crying upon waking
Intermittent muscle contraction

*DU 14
*LI 11
*Hand jing well

*SJ 18
*CV 12
*LI 4
*ST 40

*Sishencong
*PC 8
*KD 1

YINGTANG   DU 26   LV 3

Gradual onset
Emaciation
Pale complexion
Lassitude
Lethargic sleep w/open eyes
Intermittent convulsion
Cold limbs
Loose stool w/undigested food
Profuse clear urine

P= deep, weak

*BL 20, 23
*CV 12
*LV 3
*KD 2

DU 20, 24
CV 4, 6
ST 36

* SUPPLEMENTAL POINTS

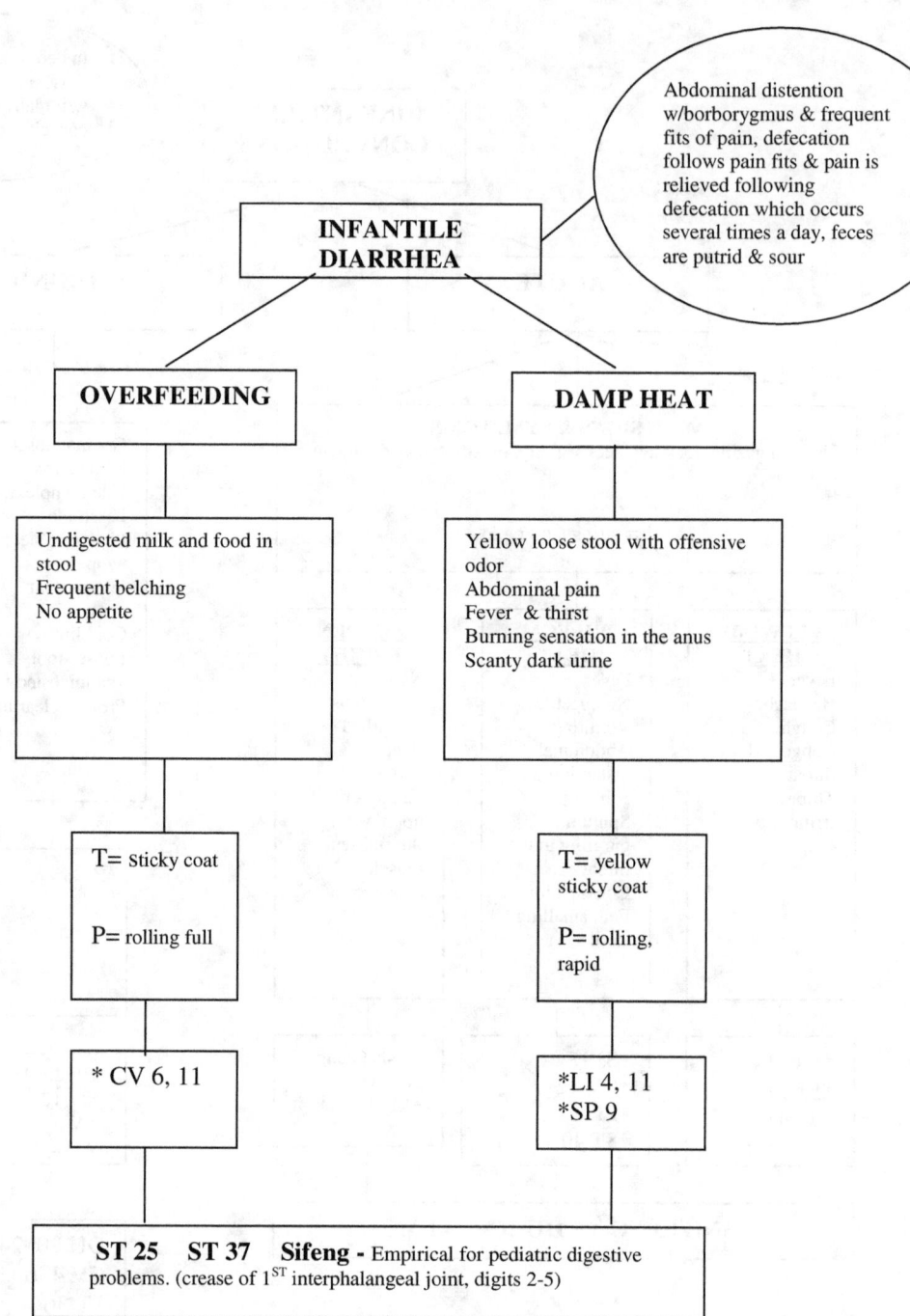

INFANTILE DIARRHEA

Abdominal distention w/borborygmus & frequent fits of pain, defecation follows pain fits & pain is relieved following defecation which occurs several times a day, feces are putrid & sour

OVERFEEDING

Undigested milk and food in stool
Frequent belching
No appetite

T= Sticky coat

P= rolling full

* CV 6, 11

DAMP HEAT

Yellow loose stool with offensive odor
Abdominal pain
Fever & thirst
Burning sensation in the anus
Scanty dark urine

T= yellow sticky coat

P= rolling, rapid

*LI 4, 11
*SP 9

ST 25   ST 37   Sifeng - Empirical for pediatric digestive problems. (crease of 1ST interphalangeal joint, digits 2-5)

* SUPPLEMENTAL POINTS

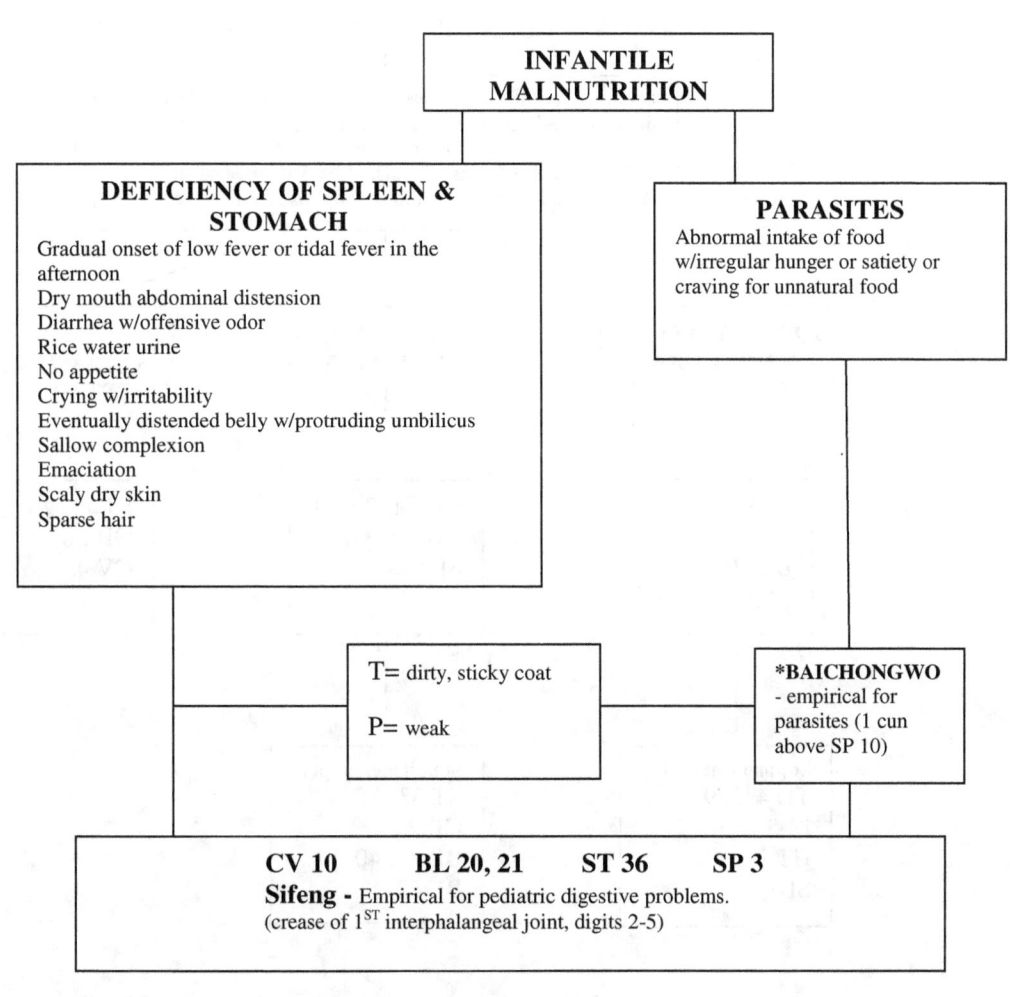

INFANTILE MALNUTRITION

DEFICIENCY OF SPLEEN & STOMACH
Gradual onset of low fever or tidal fever in the afternoon
Dry mouth abdominal distension
Diarrhea w/offensive odor
Rice water urine
No appetite
Crying w/irritability
Eventually distended belly w/protruding umbilicus
Sallow complexion
Emaciation
Scaly dry skin
Sparse hair

PARASITES
Abnormal intake of food w/irregular hunger or satiety or craving for unnatural food

T= dirty, sticky coat

P= weak

***BAICHONGWO**
- empirical for parasites (1 cun above SP 10)

CV 10   BL 20, 21   ST 36   SP 3
Sifeng - Empirical for pediatric digestive problems.
(crease of 1ST interphalangeal joint, digits 2-5)

* SUPPLEMENTAL POINTS

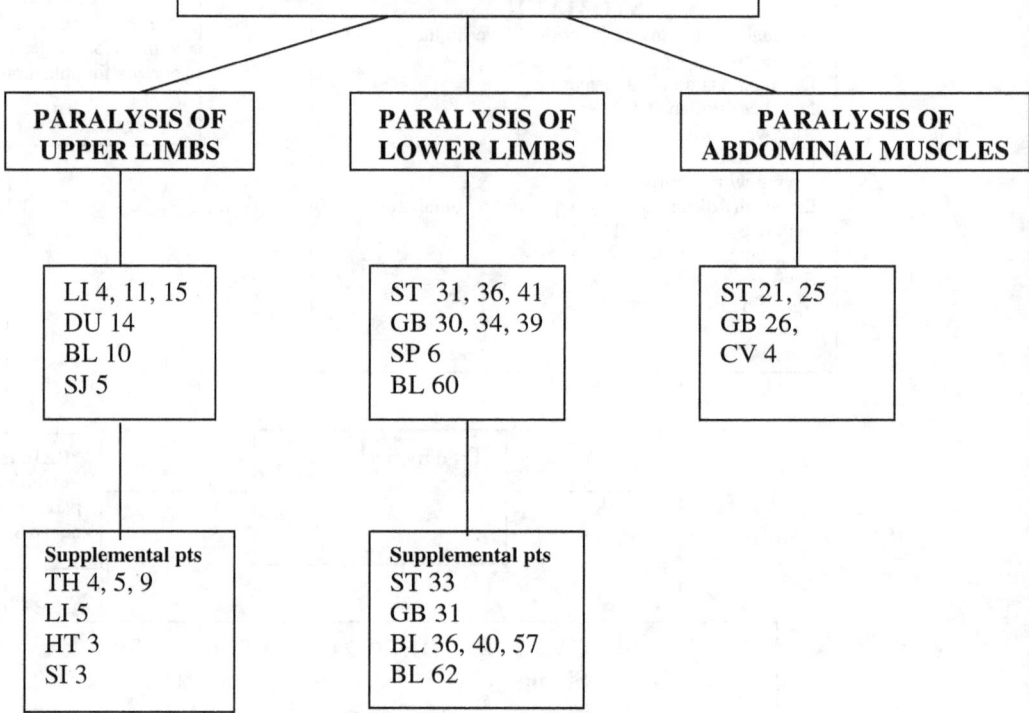

INFANTILE
PARALYSIS

Paralysis may affect any part of the body, especially the lower
limbs, w/weakness of muscles & cold skin, paralysis of
abdominal muscles is shown by abdominal bulging when
crying, in chronic cases muscular atrophy of affected areas
occurs, w/deformity of the trunk, paralysis is intractable.

PARALYSIS OF
UPPER LIMBS

PARALYSIS OF
LOWER LIMBS

PARALYSIS OF
ABDOMINAL MUSCLES

LI 4, 11, 15
DU 14
BL 10
SJ 5

ST 31, 36, 41
GB 30, 34, 39
SP 6
BL 60

ST 21, 25
GB 26,
CV 4

Supplemental pts
TH 4, 5, 9
LI 5
HT 3
SI 3

Supplemental pts
ST 33
GB 31
BL 36, 40, 57
BL 62

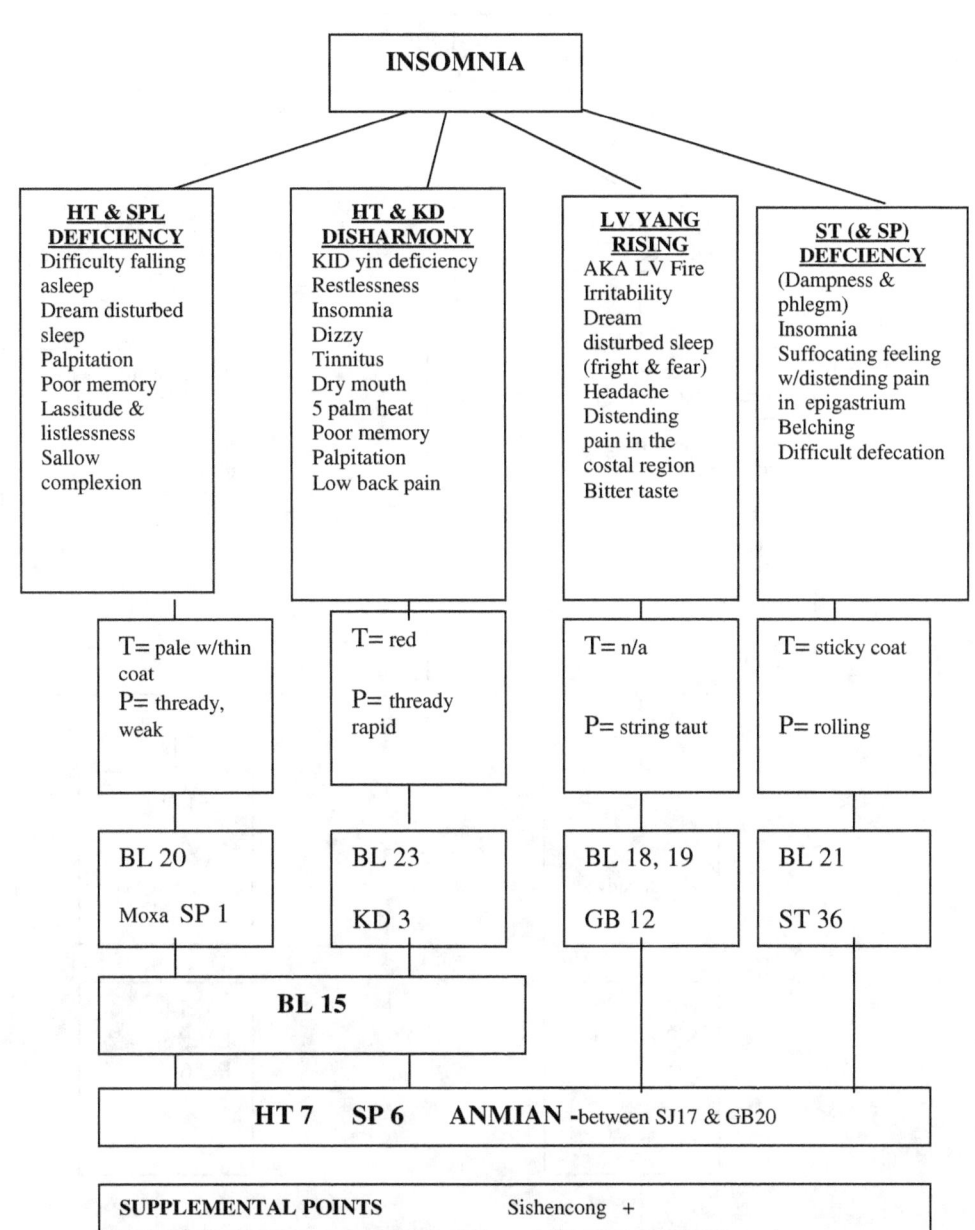

INSOMNIA

HT & SPL DEFICIENCY
Difficulty falling asleep
Dream disturbed sleep
Palpitation
Poor memory
Lassitude & listlessness
Sallow complexion

HT & KD DISHARMONY
KID yin deficiency
Restlessness
Insomnia
Dizzy
Tinnitus
Dry mouth
5 palm heat
Poor memory
Palpitation
Low back pain

LV YANG RISING
AKA LV Fire
Irritability
Dream disturbed sleep (fright & fear)
Headache
Distending pain in the costal region
Bitter taste

ST (& SP) DEFCIENCY
(Dampness & phlegm)
Insomnia
Suffocating feeling w/distending pain in epigastrium
Belching
Difficult defecation

T= pale w/thin coat
P= thready, weak

T= red
P= thready rapid

T= n/a
P= string taut

T= sticky coat
P= rolling

BL 20
Moxa SP 1

BL 23
KD 3

BL 18, 19
GB 12

BL 21
ST 36

BL 15

HT 7   SP 6   **ANMIAN** -between SJ17 & GB20

SUPPLEMENTAL POINTS   Sishencong +

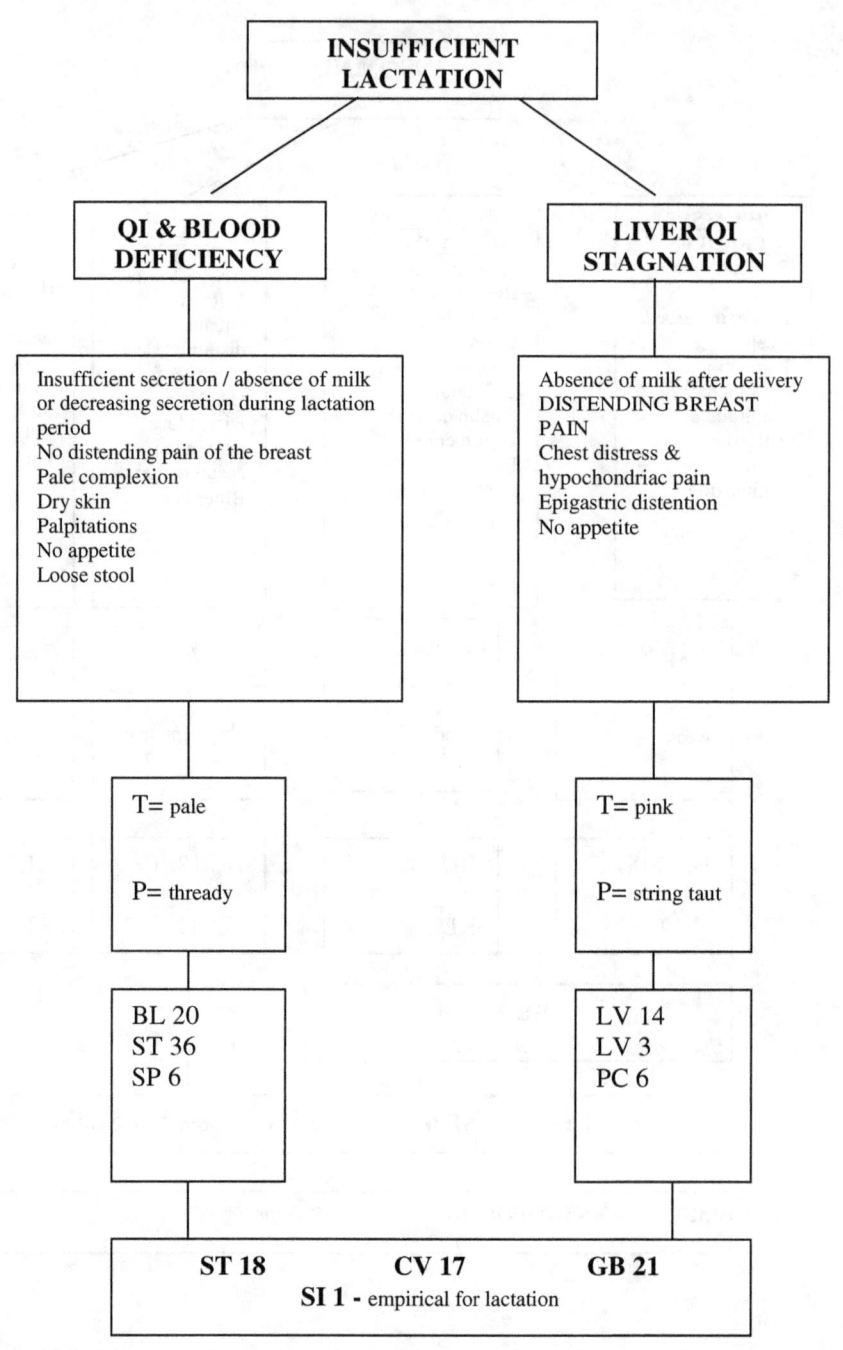

INSUFFICIENT
LACTATION

QI & BLOOD DEFICIENCY	LIVER QI STAGNATION
Insufficient secretion / absence of milk or decreasing secretion during lactation period No distending pain of the breast Pale complexion Dry skin Palpitations No appetite Loose stool	Absence of milk after delivery DISTENDING BREAST PAIN Chest distress & hypochondriac pain Epigastric distention No appetite
T= pale P= thready	T= pink P= string taut
BL 20 ST 36 SP 6	LV 14 LV 3 PC 6

ST 18   CV 17   GB 21

SI 1 - empirical for lactation

LACTIFUGE DELACTATION BL 41 & BL 37 acupuncture + moxa can suppress milk secretion

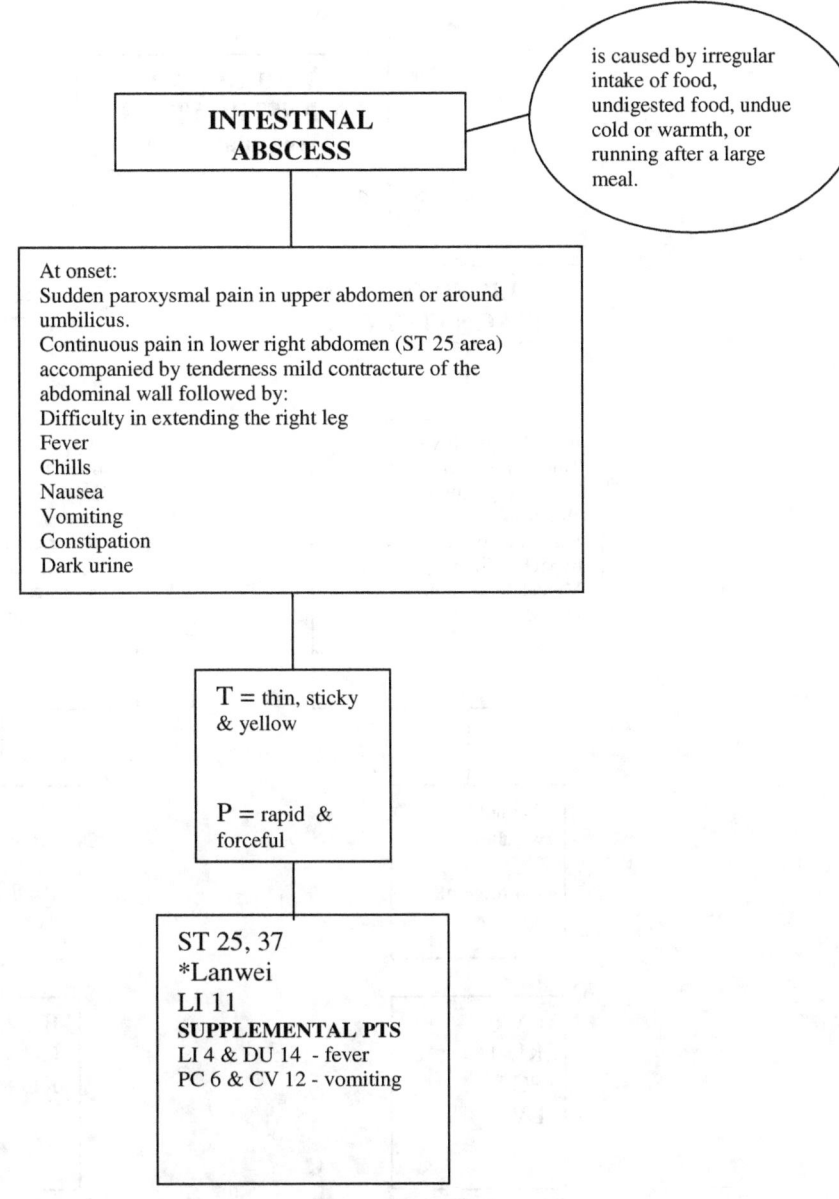

INTESTINAL ABSCESS

is caused by irregular intake of food, undigested food, undue cold or warmth, or running after a large meal.

At onset:
Sudden paroxysmal pain in upper abdomen or around umbilicus.
Continuous pain in lower right abdomen (ST 25 area) accompanied by tenderness mild contracture of the abdominal wall followed by:
Difficulty in extending the right leg
Fever
Chills
Nausea
Vomiting
Constipation
Dark urine

T = thin, sticky & yellow

P = rapid & forceful

ST 25, 37
*Lanwei
LI 11
SUPPLEMENTAL PTS
LI 4 & DU 14 - fever
PC 6 & CV 12 - vomiting

* EMPIRICAL POINT for treating intestinal abscess. The tender spot located approximately 2 cun below ST 36.

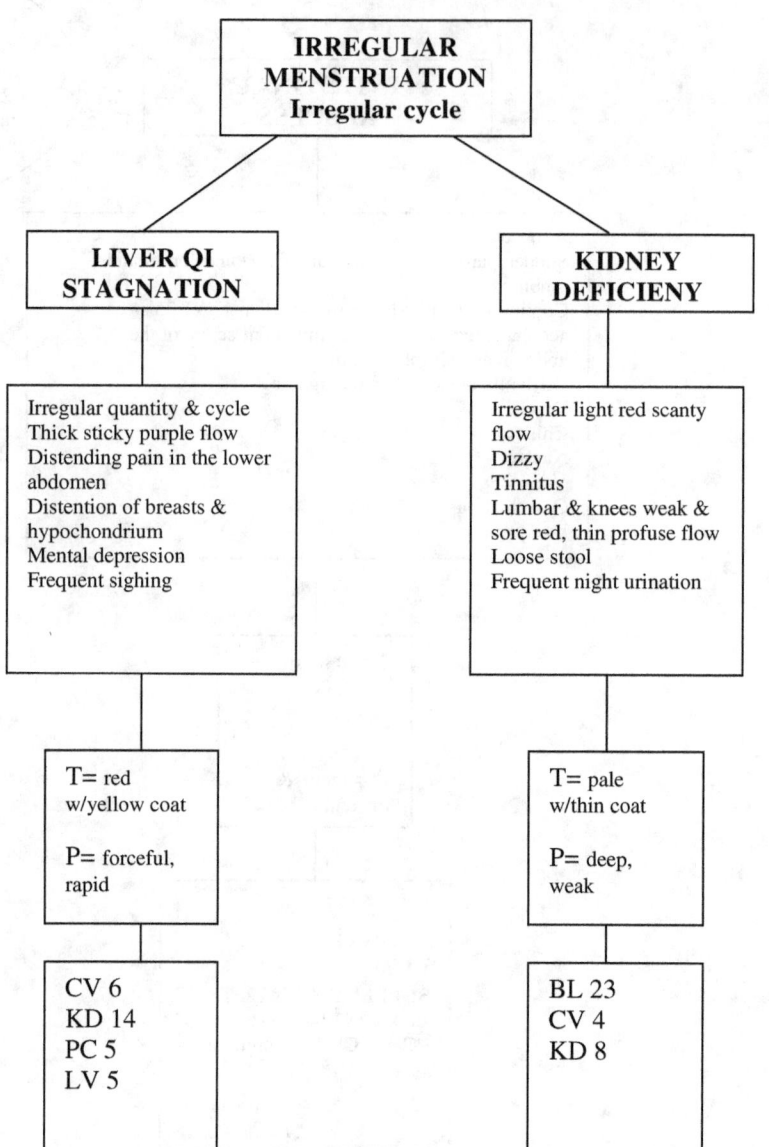

IRREGULAR MENSTRUATION
Irregular cycle

LIVER QI STAGNATION

Irregular quantity & cycle
Thick sticky purple flow
Distending pain in the lower
abdomen
Distention of breasts &
hypochondrium
Mental depression
Frequent sighing

T= red
w/yellow coat

P= forceful,
rapid

CV 6
KD 14
PC 5
LV 5

KIDNEY DEFICIENY

Irregular light red scanty
flow
Dizzy
Tinnitus
Lumbar & knees weak &
sore red, thin profuse flow
Loose stool
Frequent night urination

T= pale
w/thin coat

P= deep,
weak

BL 23
CV 4
KD 8

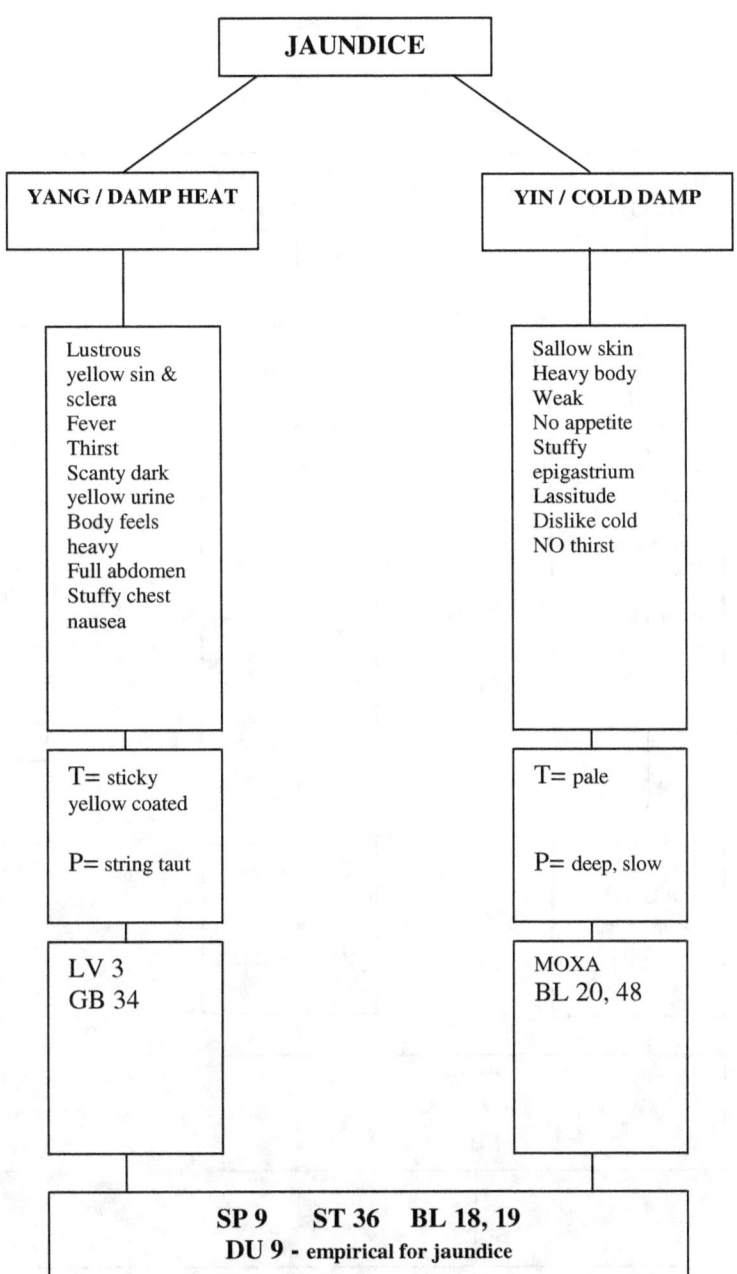

JAUNDICE

YANG / DAMP HEAT

Lustrous
yellow sin &
sclera
Fever
Thirst
Scanty dark
yellow urine
Body feels
heavy
Full abdomen
Stuffy chest
nausea

T= sticky
yellow coated

P= string taut

LV 3
GB 34

YIN / COLD DAMP

Sallow skin
Heavy body
Weak
No appetite
Stuffy
epigastrium
Lassitude
Dislike cold
NO thirst

T= pale

P= deep, slow

MOXA
BL 20, 48

SP 9   ST 36   BL 18, 19
DU 9 - empirical for jaundice

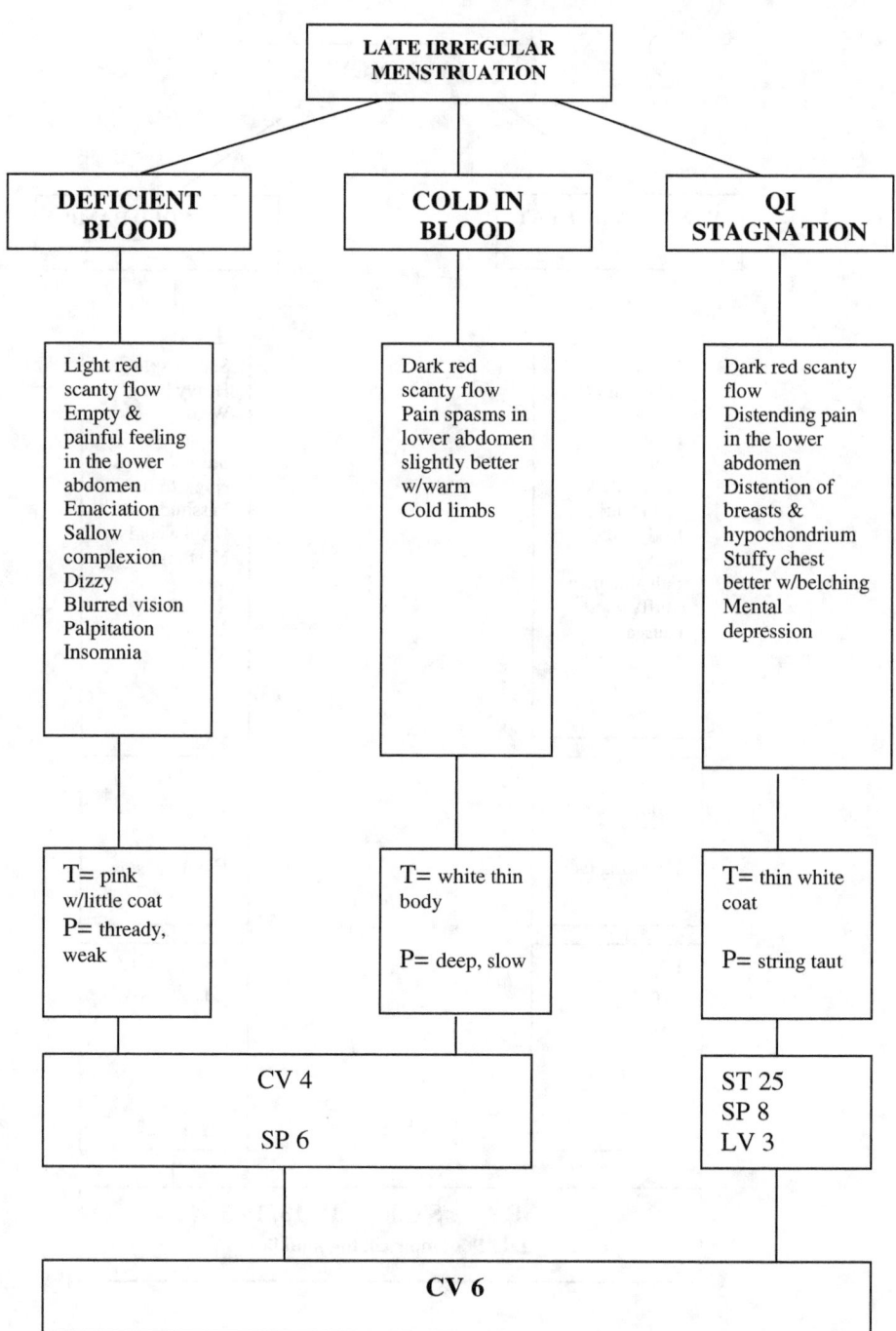

LATE IRREGULAR MENSTRUATION

DEFICIENT BLOOD

Light red scanty flow
Empty & painful feeling in the lower abdomen
Emaciation
Sallow complexion
Dizzy
Blurred vision
Palpitation
Insomnia

T= pink w/little coat
P= thready, weak

CV 4

SP 6

COLD IN BLOOD

Dark red scanty flow
Pain spasms in lower abdomen slightly better w/warm
Cold limbs

T= white thin body

P= deep, slow

QI STAGNATION

Dark red scanty flow
Distending pain in the lower abdomen
Distention of breasts & hypochondrium
Stuffy chest better w/belching
Mental depression

T= thin white coat

P= string taut

ST 25
SP 8
LV 3

CV 6

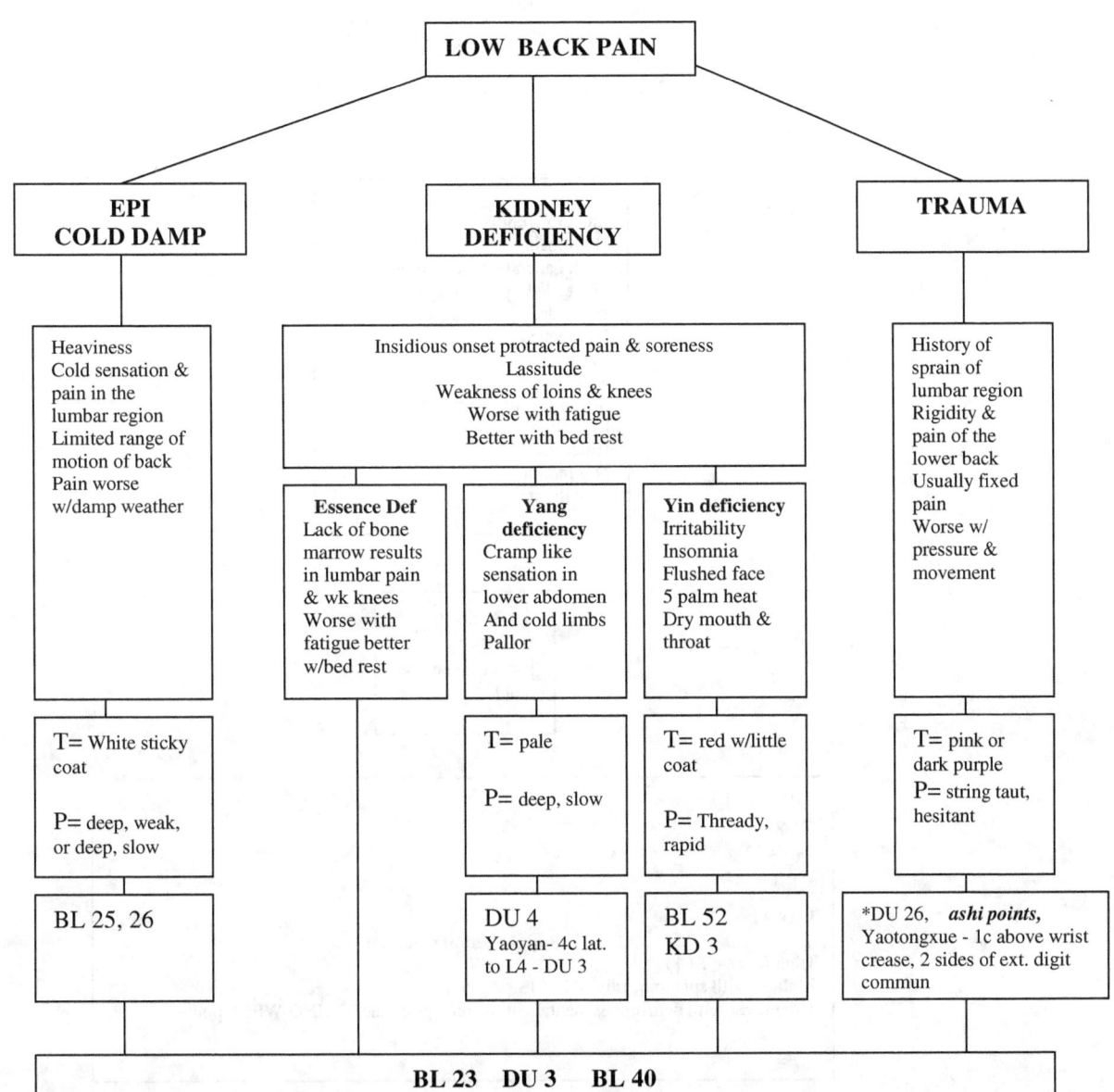

LOW BACK PAIN

EPI COLD DAMP

Heaviness
Cold sensation &
pain in the
lumbar region
Limited range of
motion of back
Pain worse
w/damp weather

T= White sticky
coat

P= deep, weak,
or deep, slow

BL 25, 26

KIDNEY DEFICIENCY

Insidious onset protracted pain & soreness
Lassitude
Weakness of loins & knees
Worse with fatigue
Better with bed rest

Essence Def
Lack of bone
marrow results
in lumbar pain
& wk knees
Worse with
fatigue better
w/bed rest

Yang deficiency
Cramp like
sensation in
lower abdomen
And cold limbs
Pallor

T= pale

P= deep, slow

DU 4
Yaoyan- 4c lat.
to L4 - DU 3

Yin deficiency
Irritability
Insomnia
Flushed face
5 palm heat
Dry mouth &
throat

T= red w/little
coat

P= Thready,
rapid

BL 52
KD 3

TRAUMA

History of
sprain of
lumbar region
Rigidity &
pain of the
lower back
Usually fixed
pain
Worse w/
pressure &
movement

T= pink or
dark purple

P= string taut,
hesitant

*DU 26, *ashi points,*
Yaotongxue - 1c above wrist
crease, 2 sides of ext. digit
commun

BL 23   DU 3   BL 40

*Empirical for lumbar

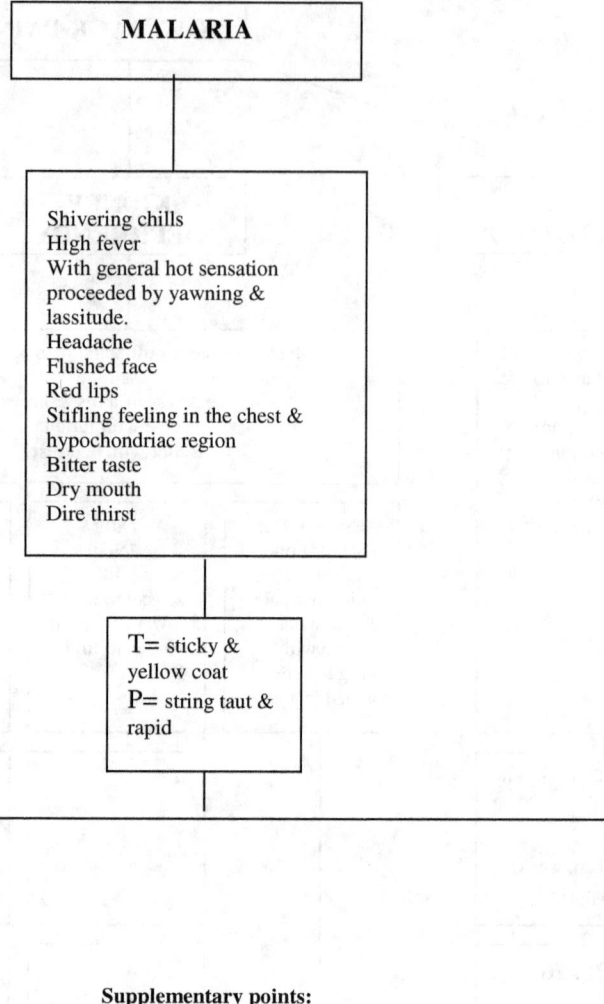

MALARIA

Shivering chills
High fever
With general hot sensation
proceeded by yawning &
lassitude.
Headache
Flushed face
Red lips
Stifling feeling in the chest &
hypochondriac region
Bitter taste
Dry mouth
Dire thirst

T= sticky &
yellow coat
P= string taut &
rapid

DU 13, 14
SI 3
PC 5
SJ 2
GB 41

Supplementary points:

High fever - LI 11
Malaria with splenomegaly - LV 13
High fever with delirium & mental confusion – prick the 12 JING WELL points.

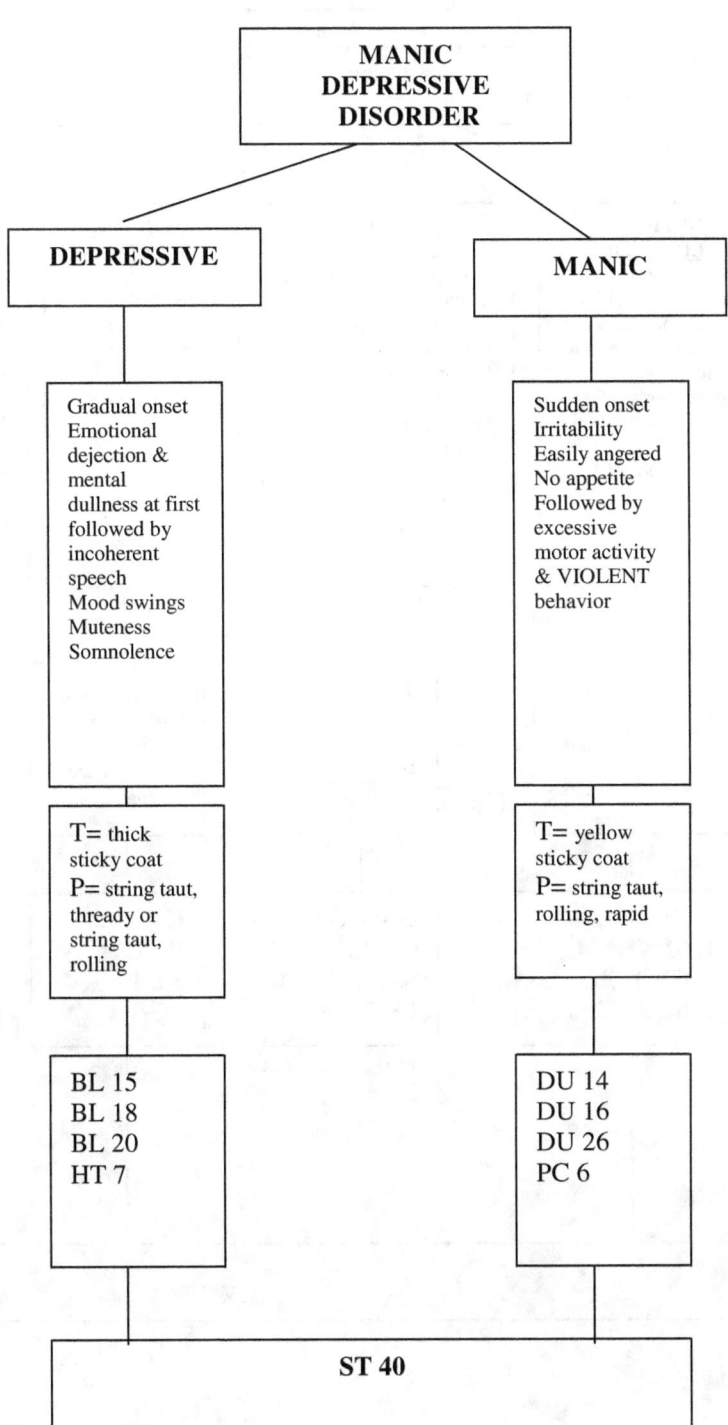

MANIC DEPRESSIVE DISORDER

DEPRESSIVE

Gradual onset
Emotional dejection & mental dullness at first followed by incoherent speech
Mood swings
Muteness
Somnolence

T= thick sticky coat
P= string taut, thready or string taut, rolling

BL 15
BL 18
BL 20
HT 7

MANIC

Sudden onset
Irritability
Easily angered
No appetite
Followed by excessive motor activity & VIOLENT behavior

T= yellow sticky coat
P= string taut, rolling, rapid

DU 14
DU 16
DU 26
PC 6

ST 40

MELANCHOLIA

is a general term used for disorders resulted from emotional depression and stagnation of qi

CONSTRAINED LIVER QI
Mental depression
Distress in the chest
Hypochondriac pain
Abdominal distention
Belching
Anorexia or
abdominal pain
Vomiting
Abnormal bowel
movement

LIVER FIRE
Headache
Dryness & bitter taste in
mouth
Irritability
Distress of the chest
Hypochondriac
distention
Acid regurgitation
Constipation
Red eyes
Tinnitus

STAGNATION OF PHLEGM
(GLOBUS
HYSTERICUS)
feeling of a lump
choking in the
throat, hard to
spit it out or to
swallow it

DEFICIENT BLOOD
(HYSTERIA)
Grief without reason
Capricious joy or anger
Suspicions
Liability to get frightened
Palpitations
Irritability
Insomnia or sudden distress of
the chest
Hiccup
Sudden aphonia
Convulsions or loss
of consciousness in severe case

T= thin sticky
coat
P= string taut

T= red with
yellow coat

P= string taut,
rapid

T= thin sticky
coat

P= string taut,
rolling

T= thin white
coat

P= string taut,
thready

BL 18
SP 4
CV 12,17
ST 36

GB 34,43
CV 13
SJ 6
LV 2

CV 17,22
PC6
ST 40

CV 14
HT 7
SP 6
SUPPLEMENTAL POINTS
PC 6, CV17 Chest distress
SP 4, CV 22 Hiccup
H 5, CV23 Sudden aphonia
LI 4, GB 34 Convulsions
DU 26, K1   Loss of
consciousness

LV 3

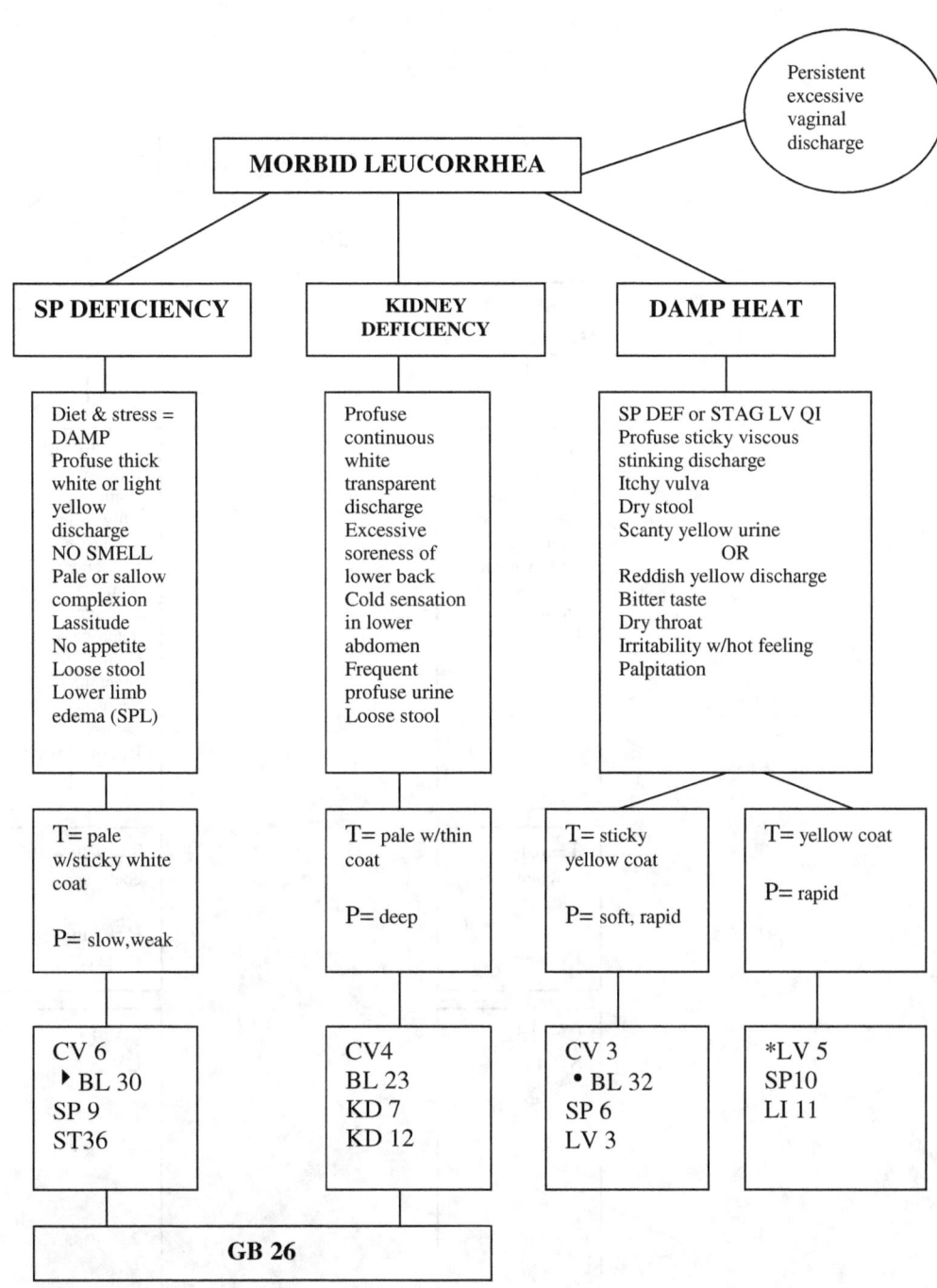

MORBID LEUCORRHEA

Persistent excessive vaginal discharge

SP DEFICIENCY

KIDNEY DEFICIENCY

DAMP HEAT

Diet & stress =
DAMP
Profuse thick
white or light
yellow
discharge
NO SMELL
Pale or sallow
complexion
Lassitude
No appetite
Loose stool
Lower limb
edema (SPL)

Profuse
continuous
white
transparent
discharge
Excessive
soreness of
lower back
Cold sensation
in lower
abdomen
Frequent
profuse urine
Loose stool

SP DEF or STAG LV QI
Profuse sticky viscous
stinking discharge
Itchy vulva
Dry stool
Scanty yellow urine
              OR
Reddish yellow discharge
Bitter taste
Dry throat
Irritability w/hot feeling
Palpitation

T= pale
w/sticky white
coat

P= slow,weak

T= pale w/thin
coat

P= deep

T= sticky
yellow coat

P= soft, rapid

T= yellow coat

P= rapid

CV 6
▶ BL 30
SP 9
ST36

CV4
BL 23
KD 7
KD 12

CV 3
• BL 32
SP 6
LV 3

*LV 5
SP10
LI 11

GB 26

• EMPIRICAL FOR LEUCORRHEA
* ITCHY VULVA
▶ EMPIRICAL FOR MORBID LEUCORRHEA

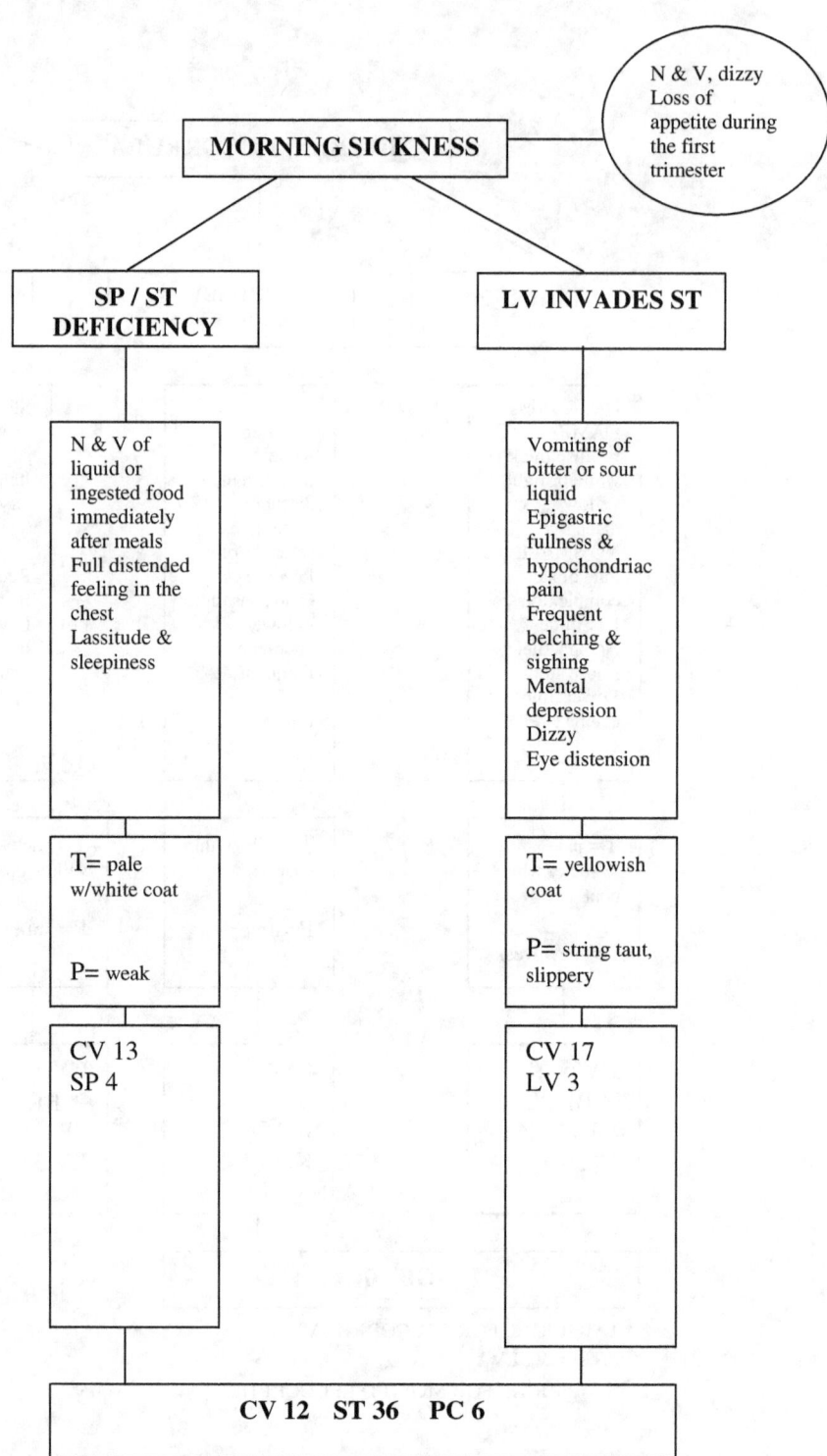

MORNING SICKNESS

N & V, dizzy
Loss of
appetite during
the first
trimester

SP / ST DEFICIENCY

LV INVADES ST

N & V of
liquid or
ingested food
immediately
after meals
Full distended
feeling in the
chest
Lassitude &
sleepiness

Vomiting of
bitter or sour
liquid
Epigastric
fullness &
hypochondriac
pain
Frequent
belching &
sighing
Mental
depression
Dizzy
Eye distension

T= pale
w/white coat

P= weak

T= yellowish
coat

P= string taut,
slippery

CV 13
SP 4

CV 17
LV 3

CV 12   ST 36   PC 6

MUMPS

Chills & fever at onset
Redness, pain & swelling in
unilateral or bilateral parotid (near
the ear) region
Difficulty chewing
If pathogenic heat is intense, the
above symptoms are accompanied
by pain & swelling in the testes,
high fever w/irritability, dry mouth,
constipation, dark urine.

T= yellow coat

P= rapid

SJ 5, 17
ST 6
LI 4, 11

SUPPLEMENTAL PTS
LU 7
DU 14
12 JING WELL PTS HAND
LV 3, 8

THICK & STICKY
NASAL DISCHARGE
(RHINORRHEA)

Nasal obstruction
Loss of sense of
smell
Thick & sticky
yellow fetid
nasal discharge
accompanied by
cough
Dull pain in
forehead

T= red w/thin
white sticky coat

P= rapid

LU 7

LI 4, 20

BITONG - at the highest pt of
the nasolabial groove.

YINTANG- midway between
the medial ends of the two
eyebrows

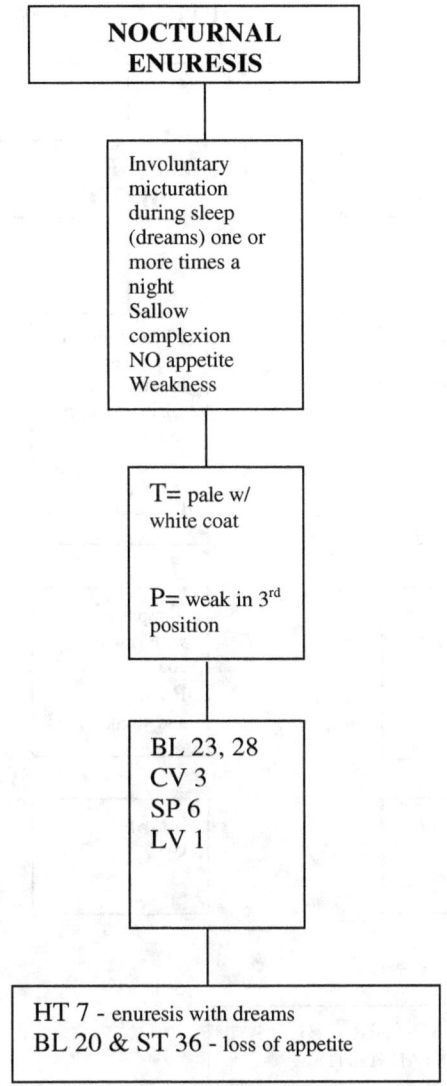

NOCTURNAL ENURESIS

Involuntary micturation during sleep (dreams) one or more times a night
Sallow complexion
NO appetite
Weakness

T= pale w/ white coat

P= weak in 3rd position

BL 23, 28
CV 3
SP 6
LV 1

HT 7 - enuresis with dreams
BL 20 & ST 36 - loss of appetite

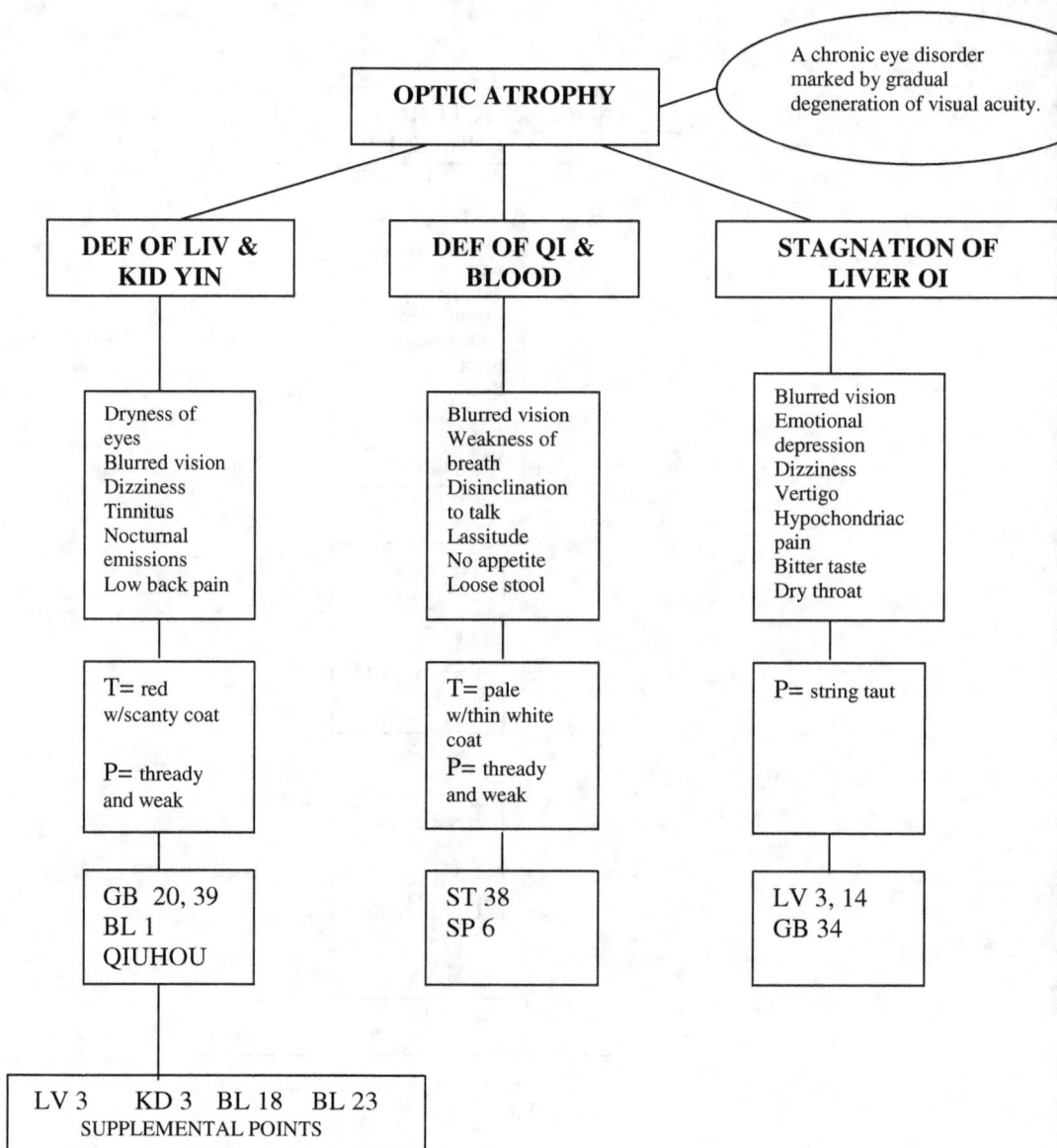

OPTIC ATROPHY

A chronic eye disorder marked by gradual degeneration of visual acuity.

DEF OF LIV & KID YIN

Dryness of eyes
Blurred vision
Dizziness
Tinnitus
Nocturnal emissions
Low back pain

T= red w/scanty coat

P= thready and weak

GB 20, 39
BL 1
QIUHOU

DEF OF QI & BLOOD

Blurred vision
Weakness of breath
Disinclination to talk
Lassitude
No appetite
Loose stool

T= pale w/thin white coat
P= thready and weak

ST 38
SP 6

STAGNATION OF LIVER OI

Blurred vision
Emotional depression
Dizziness
Vertigo
Hypochondriac pain
Bitter taste
Dry throat

P= string taut

LV 3, 14
GB 34

LV 3   KD 3   BL 18   BL 23
SUPPLEMENTAL POINTS

PALPITATIONS

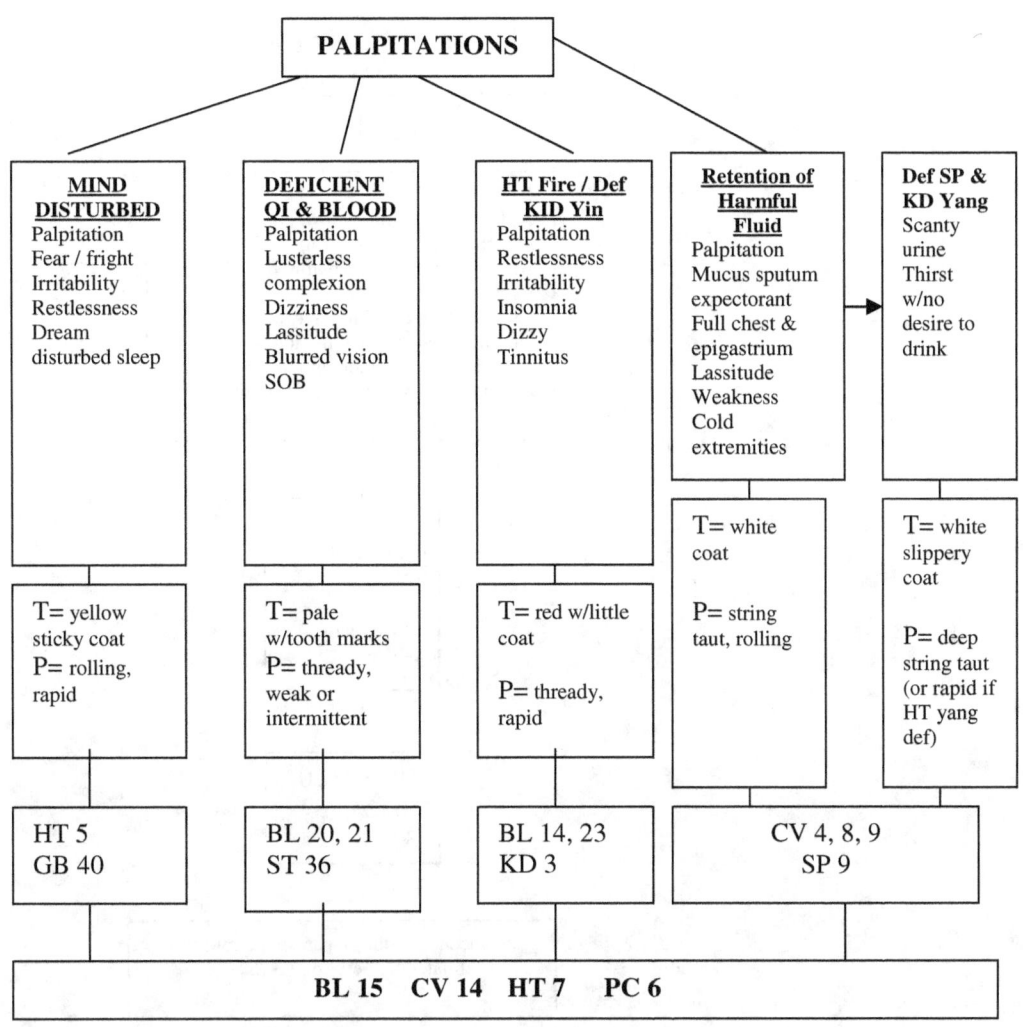

MIND DISTURBED	DEFICIENT QI & BLOOD	HT Fire / Def KID Yin	Retention of Harmful Fluid	Def SP & KD Yang
Palpitation Fear / fright Irritability Restlessness Dream disturbed sleep	Palpitation Lusterless complexion Dizziness Lassitude Blurred vision SOB	Palpitation Restlessness Irritability Insomnia Dizzy Tinnitus	Palpitation Mucus sputum expectorant Full chest & epigastrium Lassitude Weakness Cold extremities	Scanty urine Thirst w/no desire to drink
T= yellow sticky coat P= rolling, rapid	T= pale w/tooth marks P= thready, weak or intermittent	T= red w/little coat P= thready, rapid	T= white coat P= string taut, rolling	T= white slippery coat P= deep string taut (or rapid if HT yang def)
HT 5 GB 40	BL 20, 21 ST 36	BL 14, 23 KD 3	CV 4, 8, 9 SP 9	

BL 15   CV 14   HT 7   PC 6

PROLAPSE OF RECTUM

SLOW onset
At first only a pulling down, distending
sensation at the anus during defecation,
which returns to normal after bowel
movement
Untreated the condition may become
chronic, evoked by slight fatigue &
requiring manual intervention; sometimes
accompanied by lassitude, weak limbs,
sallow complexion, dizzy, palpitation.

T= pale w/
white coat

P= thready,
feeble

DU 1 & 20
BL 25
ST 36

cutaneous needling - paraspinal muscles
bilaterally between L3 & S2

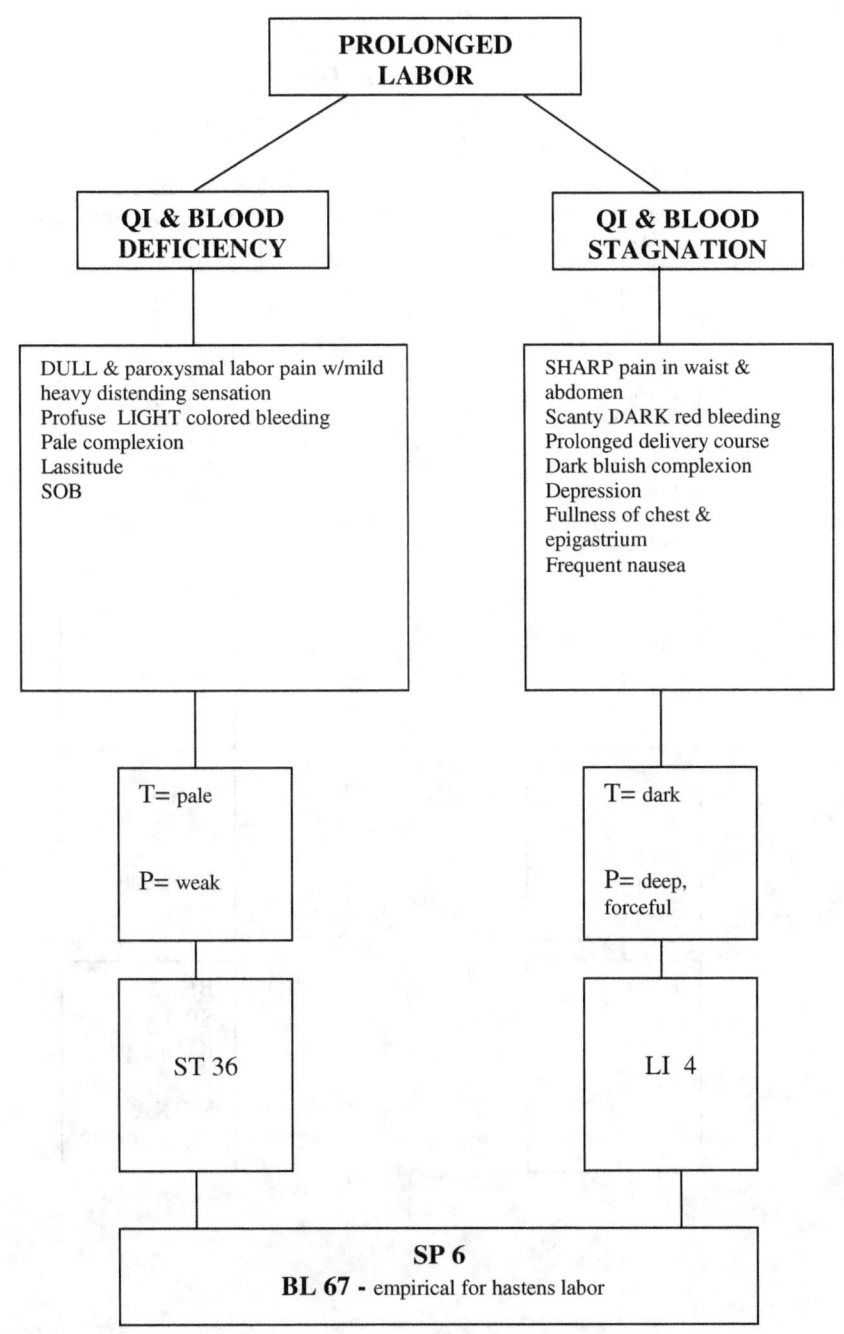

PROLONGED LABOR

QI & BLOOD DEFICIENCY

QI & BLOOD STAGNATION

DULL & paroxysmal labor pain w/mild heavy distending sensation
Profuse LIGHT colored bleeding
Pale complexion
Lassitude
SOB

SHARP pain in waist & abdomen
Scanty DARK red bleeding
Prolonged delivery course
Dark bluish complexion
Depression
Fullness of chest & epigastrium
Frequent nausea

T= pale

P= weak

T= dark

P= deep, forceful

ST 36

LI 4

SP 6
BL 67 - empirical for hastens labor

MALPOSITION OF FETUS BL 67 bilateral with moxa once or twice daily until position is corrected

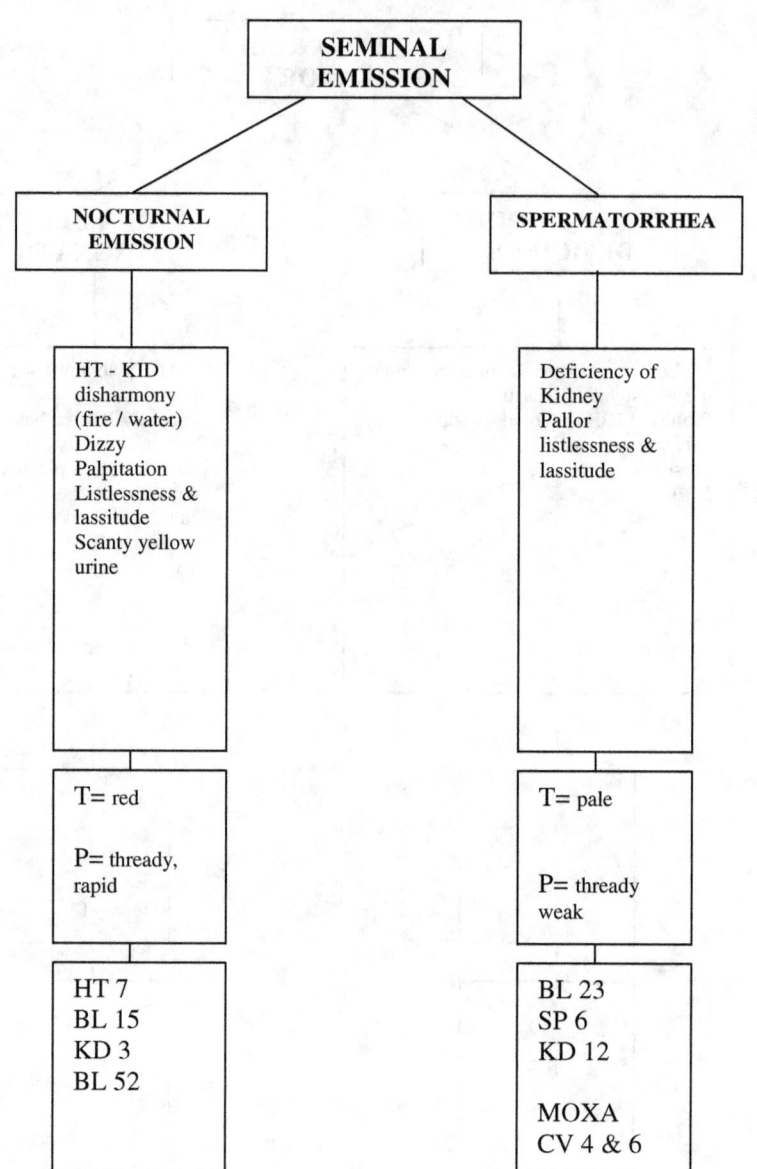

SEMINAL
EMISSION

NOCTURNAL
EMISSION

SPERMATORRHEA

HT - KID
disharmony
(fire / water)
Dizzy
Palpitation
Listlessness &
lassitude
Scanty yellow
urine

Deficiency of
Kidney
Pallor
listlessness &
lassitude

T= red

P= thready,
rapid

T= pale

P= thready
weak

HT 7
BL 15
KD 3
BL 52

BL 23
SP 6
KD 12

MOXA
CV 4 & 6

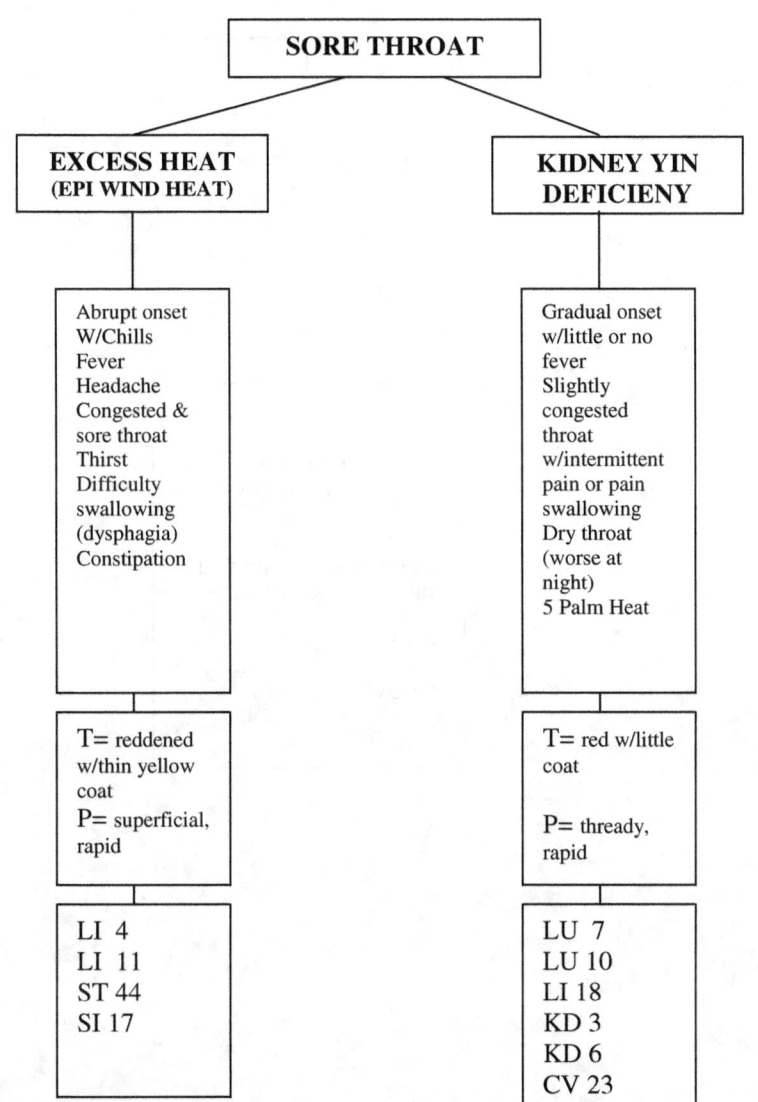

SORE THROAT

EXCESS HEAT
(EPI WIND HEAT)

KIDNEY YIN
DEFICIENY

Abrupt onset W/Chills Fever Headache Congested & sore throat Thirst Difficulty swallowing (dysphagia) Constipation	Gradual onset w/little or no fever Slightly congested throat w/intermittent pain or pain swallowing Dry throat (worse at night) 5 Palm Heat
T= reddened w/thin yellow coat P= superficial, rapid	T= red w/little coat P= thready, rapid
LI 4 LI 11 ST 44 SI 17	LU 7 LU 10 LI 18 KD 3 KD 6 CV 23

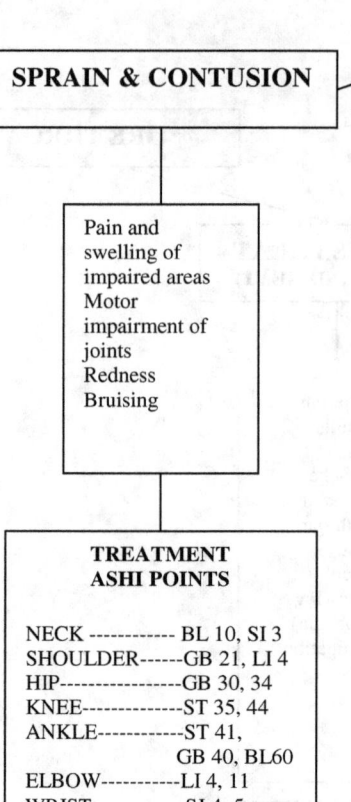

SPRAIN & CONTUSION

Injury of soft tissue such as skin muscles & tendons of trunk or limbs w/o fracture, dislocation or wound

Pain and swelling of impaired areas
Motor impairment of joints
Redness
Bruising

TREATMENT
ASHI POINTS

NECK ------------ BL 10, SI 3
SHOULDER------GB 21, LI 4
HIP-----------------GB 30, 34
KNEE--------------ST 35, 44
ANKLE------------ST 41,
                 GB 40, BL60
ELBOW-----------LI 4, 11
WRIST-------------SJ 4, 5

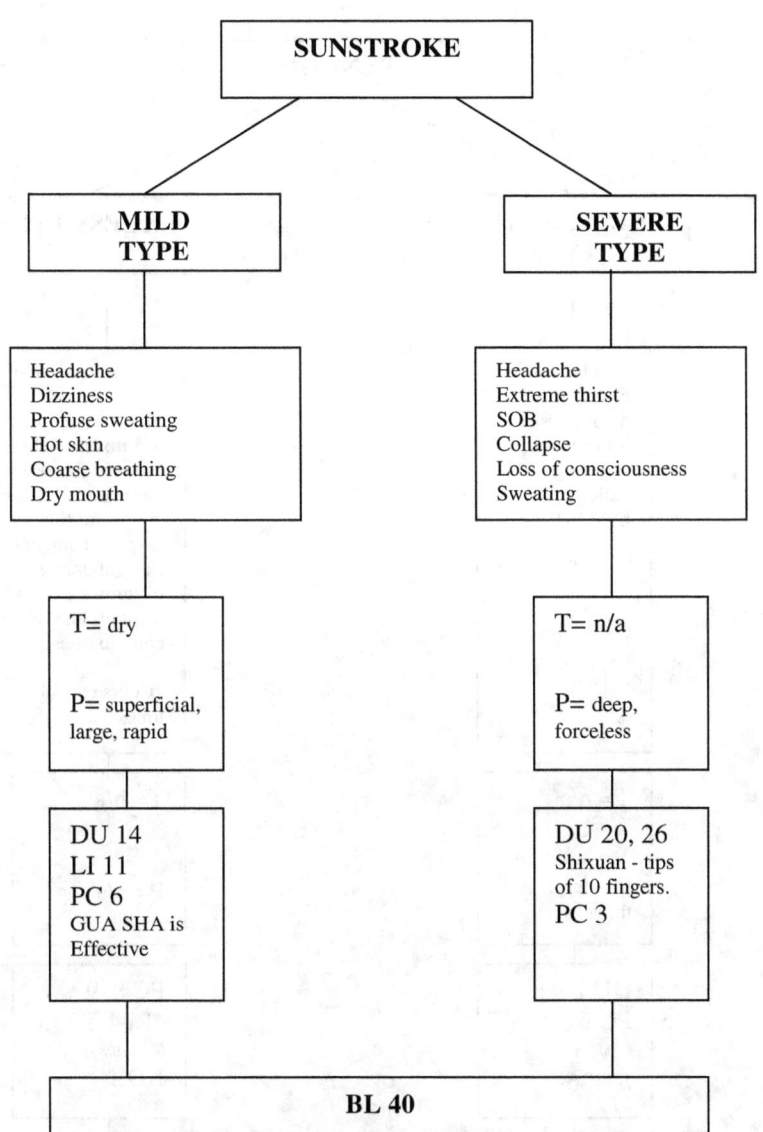

SUNSTROKE

MILD TYPE

Headache
Dizziness
Profuse sweating
Hot skin
Coarse breathing
Dry mouth

T= dry

P= superficial, large, rapid

DU 14
LI 11
PC 6
GUA SHA is
Effective

SEVERE TYPE

Headache
Extreme thirst
SOB
Collapse
Loss of consciousness
Sweating

T= n/a

P= deep, forceless

DU 20, 26
Shixuan - tips
of 10 fingers.
PC 3

BL 40

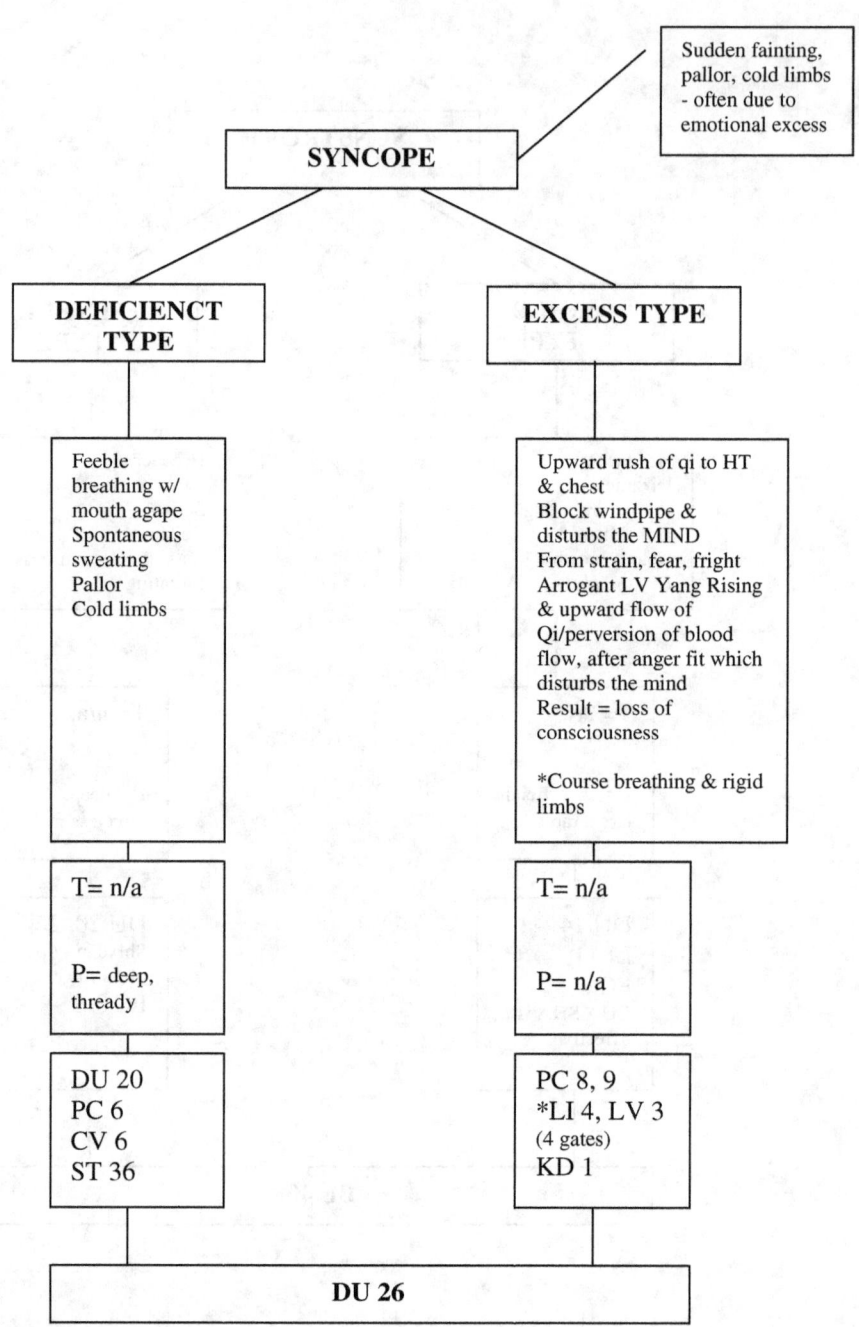

SYNCOPE

Sudden fainting, pallor, cold limbs - often due to emotional excess

DEFICIENCT TYPE

EXCESS TYPE

Feeble breathing w/ mouth agape
Spontaneous sweating
Pallor
Cold limbs

Upward rush of qi to HT & chest
Block windpipe & disturbs the MIND
From strain, fear, fright
Arrogant LV Yang Rising & upward flow of Qi/perversion of blood flow, after anger fit which disturbs the mind
Result = loss of consciousness

*Course breathing & rigid limbs

T= n/a

P= deep, thready

T= n/a

P= n/a

DU 20
PC 6
CV 6
ST 36

PC 8, 9
*LI 4, LV 3
(4 gates)
KD 1

DU 26

DISTINGUISH SYNCOPE FROM:
WIND STROKE - loss of consciousness with hemiplegia & deviated mouth; often sequela after regaining consciousness.
EPILEPSY - loss of consciousness w/convulsions, frothy saliva or yelling: client normal after regaining consciousness.

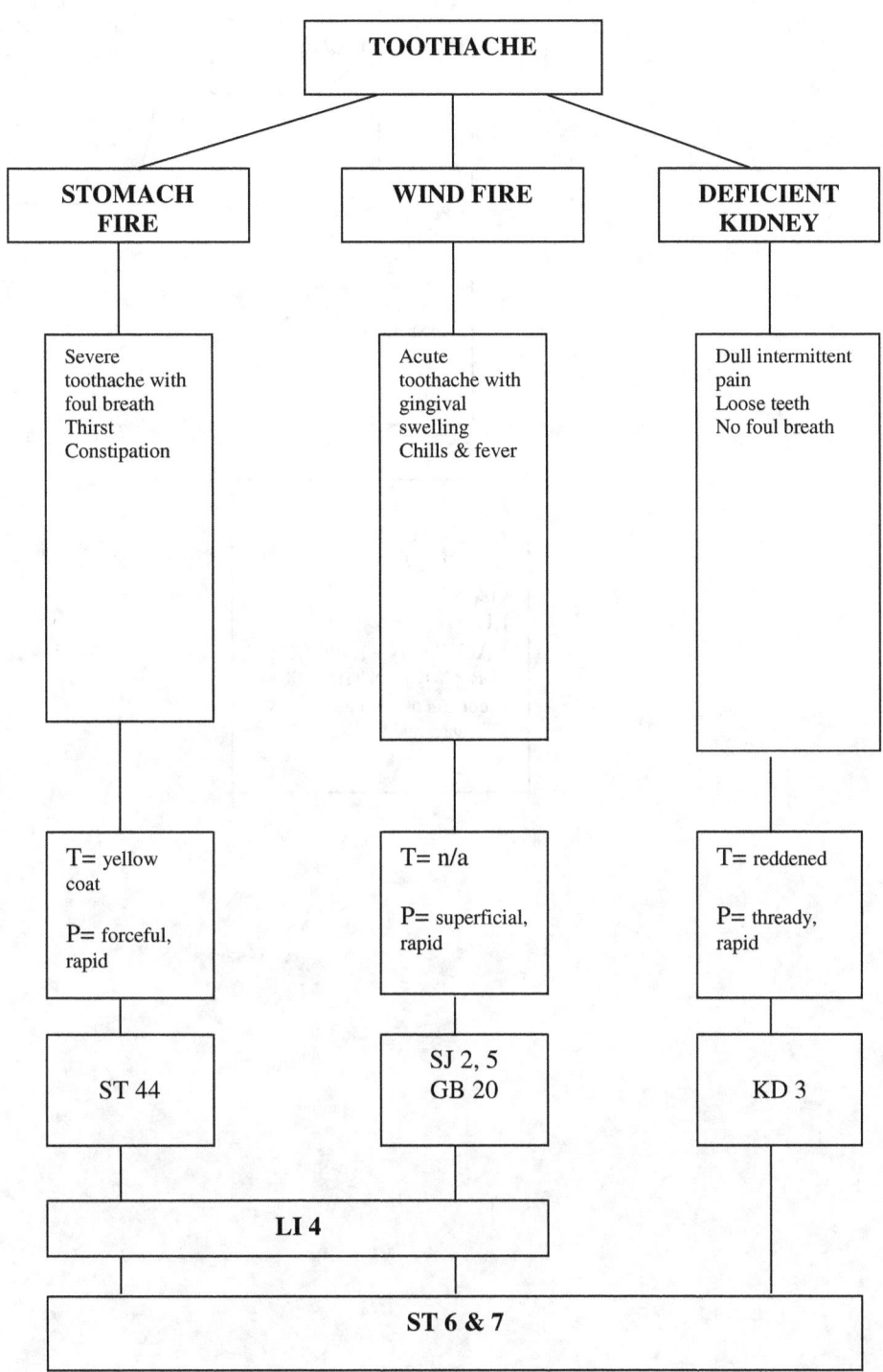

TOOTHACHE

STOMACH FIRE

WIND FIRE

DEFICIENT KIDNEY

Severe toothache with foul breath
Thirst
Constipation

Acute toothache with gingival swelling
Chills & fever

Dull intermittent pain
Loose teeth
No foul breath

T= yellow coat

P= forceful, rapid

T= n/a

P= superficial, rapid

T= reddened

P= thready, rapid

ST 44

SJ 2, 5
GB 20

KD 3

LI 4

ST 6 & 7

TORTICOLLIS

A wry neck caused by awkward sleeping posture or attack of wind cold on nape of neck that leads to disturbance of local circulation of qi in the meridians.

Stiffness
Pain of the neck & nape
Wry neck towards one side w/motor impairment

DU 14
BL 10, 60
SI 3, 7, 14
GB 39
LU 7
LAOZHEN - EMPIRICAL FOR CRICK IN THE NECK - (dorsum of hand btwn 2nd & 3rd metacarpal bones.)

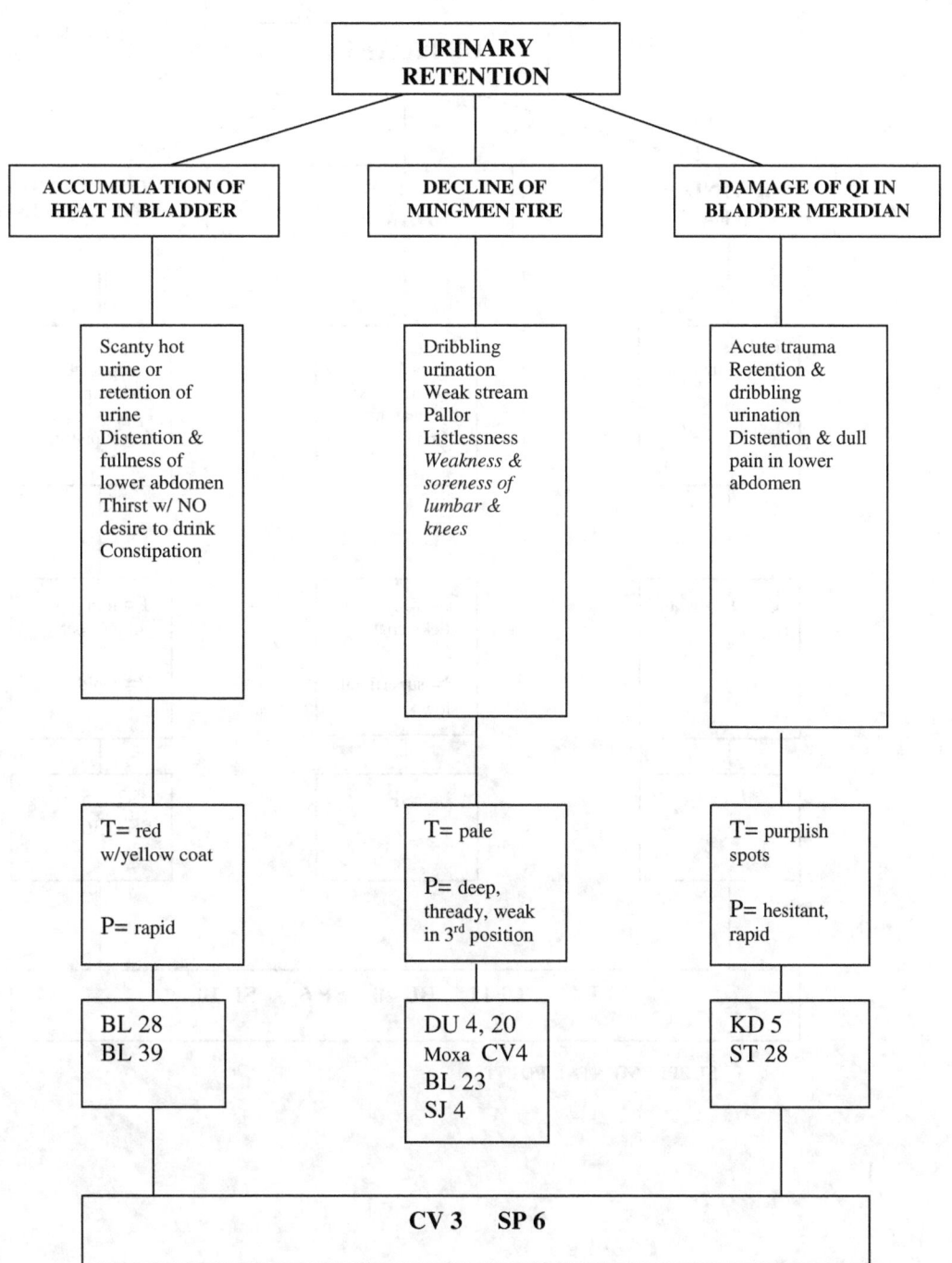

URINARY RETENTION

ACCUMULATION OF HEAT IN BLADDER

Scanty hot urine or retention of urine
Distention & fullness of lower abdomen
Thirst w/ NO desire to drink
Constipation

T= red w/yellow coat

P= rapid

BL 28
BL 39

DECLINE OF MINGMEN FIRE

Dribbling urination
Weak stream
Pallor
Listlessness
Weakness & soreness of lumbar & knees

T= pale

P= deep, thready, weak in 3rd position

DU 4, 20
Moxa CV4
BL 23
SJ 4

DAMAGE OF QI IN BLADDER MERIDIAN

Acute trauma
Retention & dribbling urination
Distention & dull pain in lower abdomen

T= purplish spots

P= hesitant, rapid

KD 5
ST 28

CV 3   SP 6

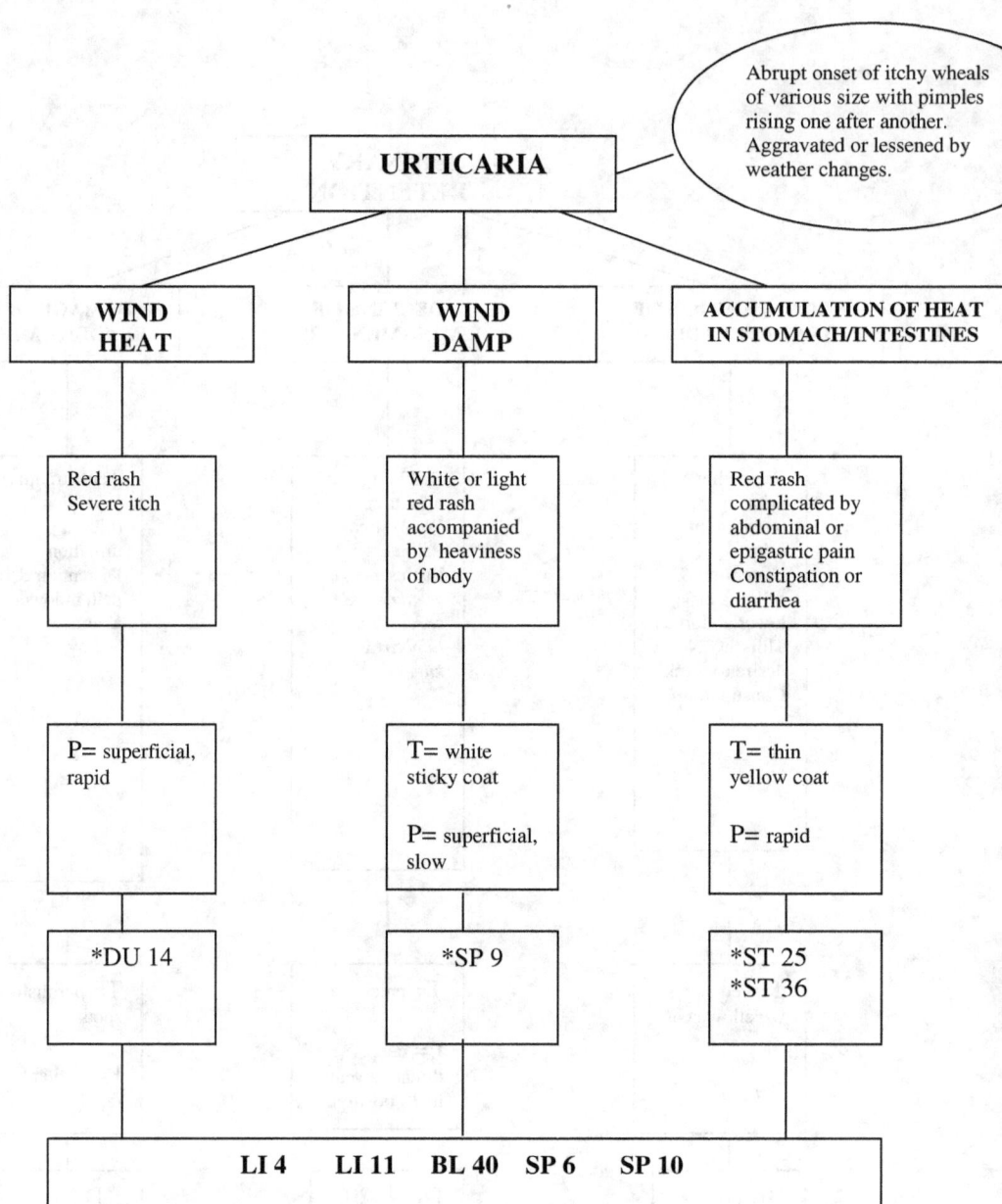

URTICARIA

Abrupt onset of itchy wheals of various size with pimples rising one after another. Aggravated or lessened by weather changes.

WIND HEAT

WIND DAMP

ACCUMULATION OF HEAT IN STOMACH/INTESTINES

Red rash
Severe itch

White or light red rash accompanied by heaviness of body

Red rash complicated by abdominal or epigastric pain Constipation or diarrhea

P= superficial, rapid

T= white sticky coat

P= superficial, slow

T= thin yellow coat

P= rapid

*DU 14

*SP 9

*ST 25
*ST 36

LI 4   LI 11   BL 40   SP 6   SP 10

*SUPPLEMENTAL POINTS

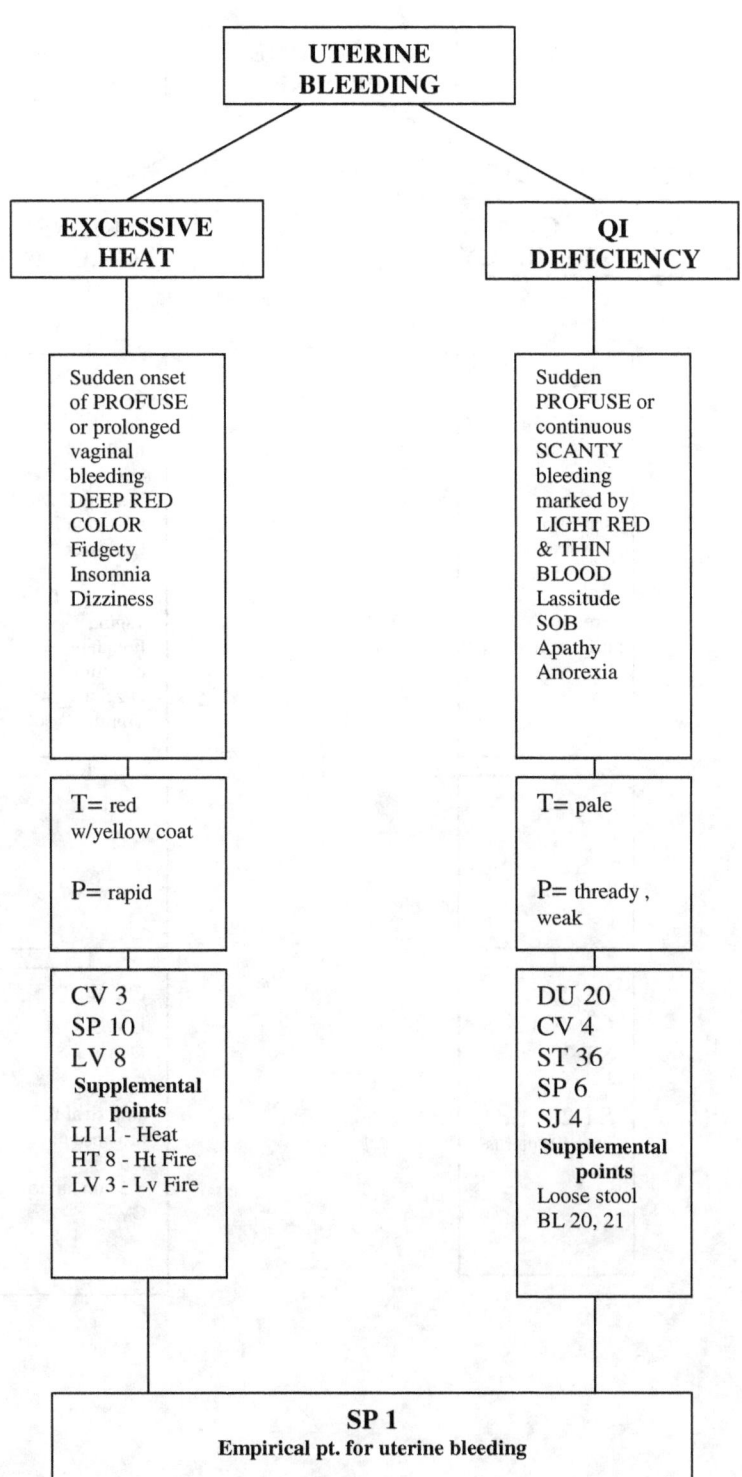

UTERINE
BLEEDING

EXCESSIVE
HEAT

QI
DEFICIENCY

Sudden onset
of PROFUSE
or prolonged
vaginal
bleeding
DEEP RED
COLOR
Fidgety
Insomnia
Dizziness

Sudden
PROFUSE or
continuous
SCANTY
bleeding
marked by
LIGHT RED
& THIN
BLOOD
Lassitude
SOB
Apathy
Anorexia

T= red
w/yellow coat

P= rapid

T= pale

P= thready ,
weak

CV 3
SP 10
LV 8
**Supplemental
points**
LI 11 - Heat
HT 8 - Ht Fire
LV 3 - Lv Fire

DU 20
CV 4
ST 36
SP 6
SJ 4
**Supplemental
points**
Loose stool
BL 20, 21

SP 1
Empirical pt. for uterine bleeding

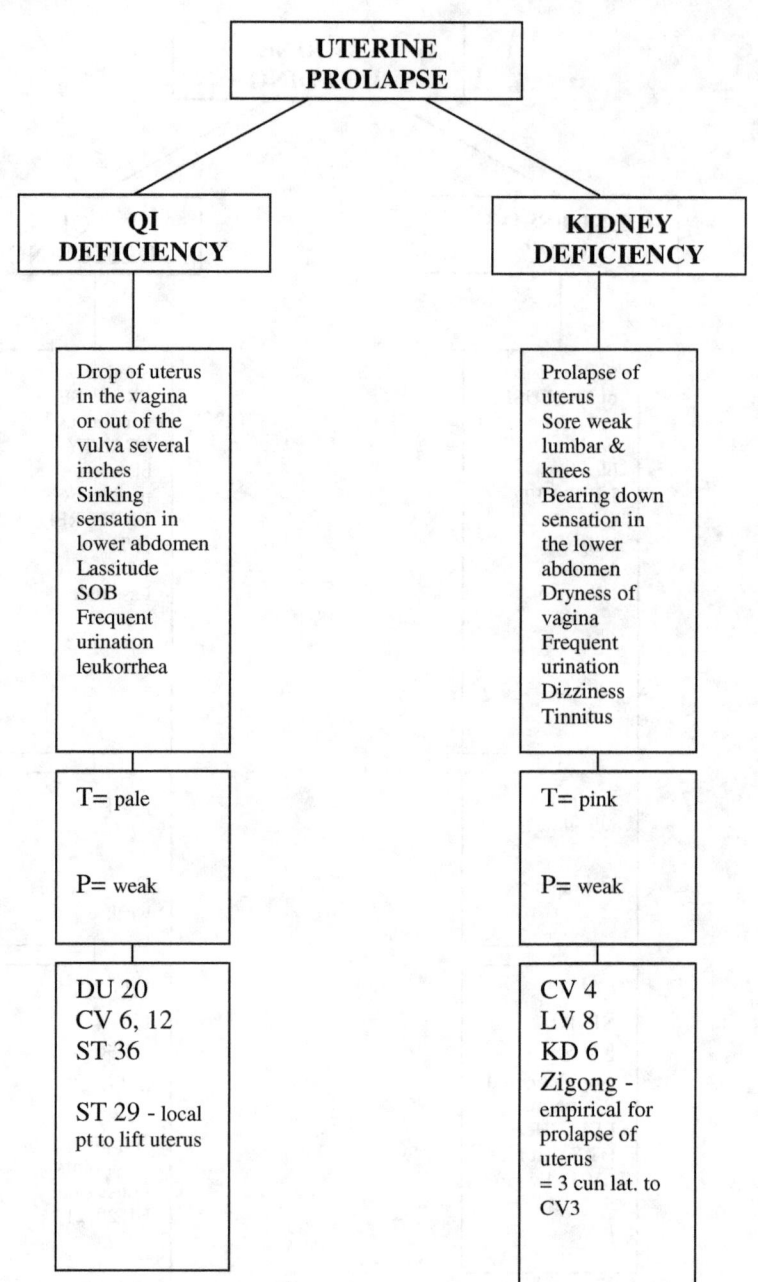

UTERINE
PROLAPSE

QI
DEFICIENCY

KIDNEY
DEFICIENCY

Drop of uterus
in the vagina
or out of the
vulva several
inches
Sinking
sensation in
lower abdomen
Lassitude
SOB
Frequent
urination
leukorrhea

Prolapse of
uterus
Sore weak
lumbar &
knees
Bearing down
sensation in
the lower
abdomen
Dryness of
vagina
Frequent
urination
Dizziness
Tinnitus

T= pale

P= weak

T= pink

P= weak

DU 20
CV 6, 12
ST 36

ST 29 - local
pt to lift uterus

CV 4
LV 8
KD 6
Zigong -
empirical for
prolapse of
uterus
= 3 cun lat. to
CV3

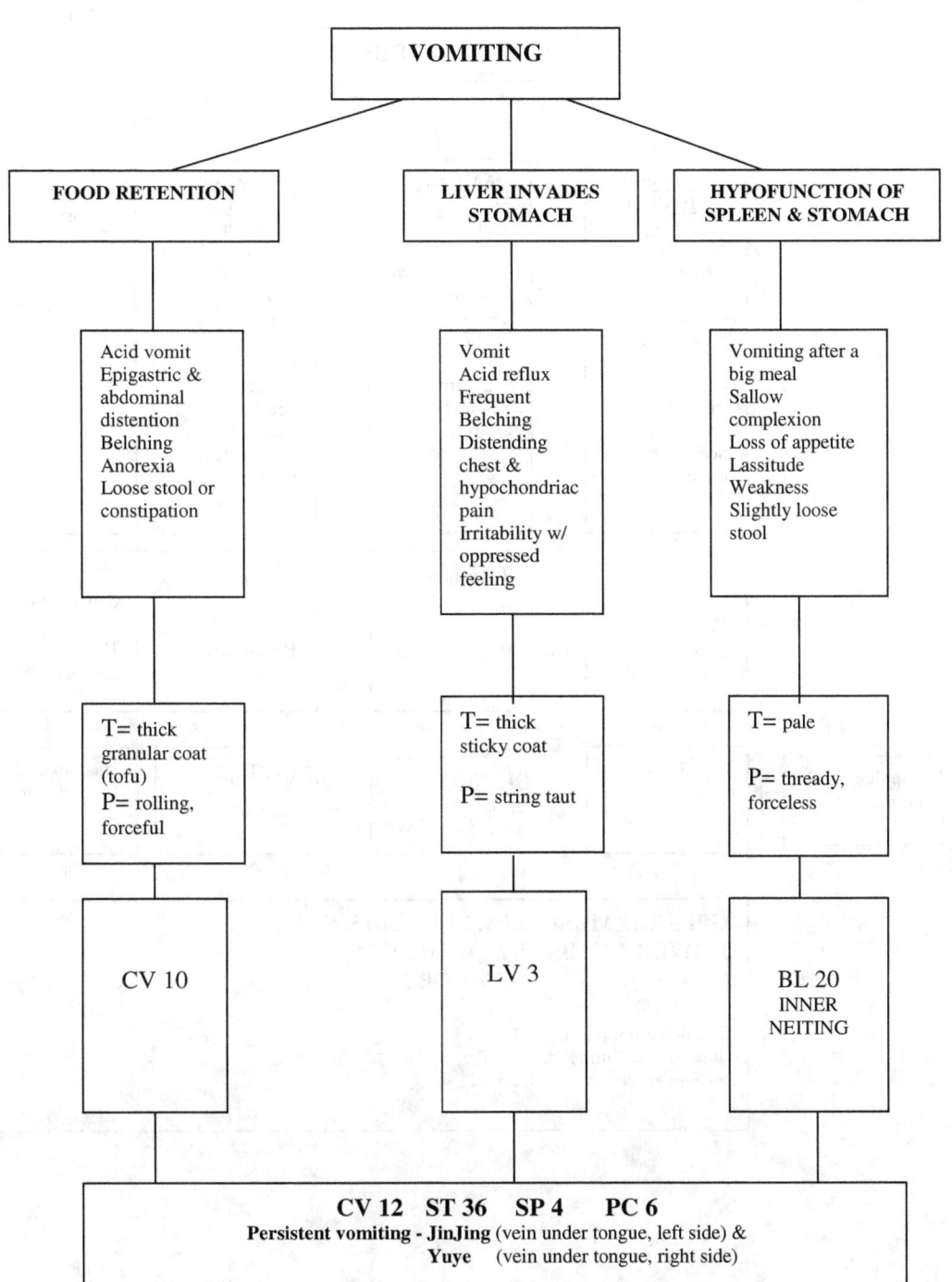

VOMITING

FOOD RETENTION

LIVER INVADES STOMACH

HYPOFUNCTION OF SPLEEN & STOMACH

Acid vomit
Epigastric &
abdominal
distention
Belching
Anorexia
Loose stool or
constipation

Vomit
Acid reflux
Frequent
Belching
Distending
chest &
hypochondriac
pain
Irritability w/
oppressed
feeling

Vomiting after a
big meal
Sallow
complexion
Loss of appetite
Lassitude
Weakness
Slightly loose
stool

T= thick
granular coat
(tofu)
P= rolling,
forceful

T= thick
sticky coat

P= string taut

T= pale

P= thready,
forceless

CV 10

LV 3

BL 20
INNER
NEITING

CV 12   ST 36   SP 4   PC 6
Persistent vomiting - **JinJing** (vein under tongue, left side) &
Yuye   (vein under tongue, right side)

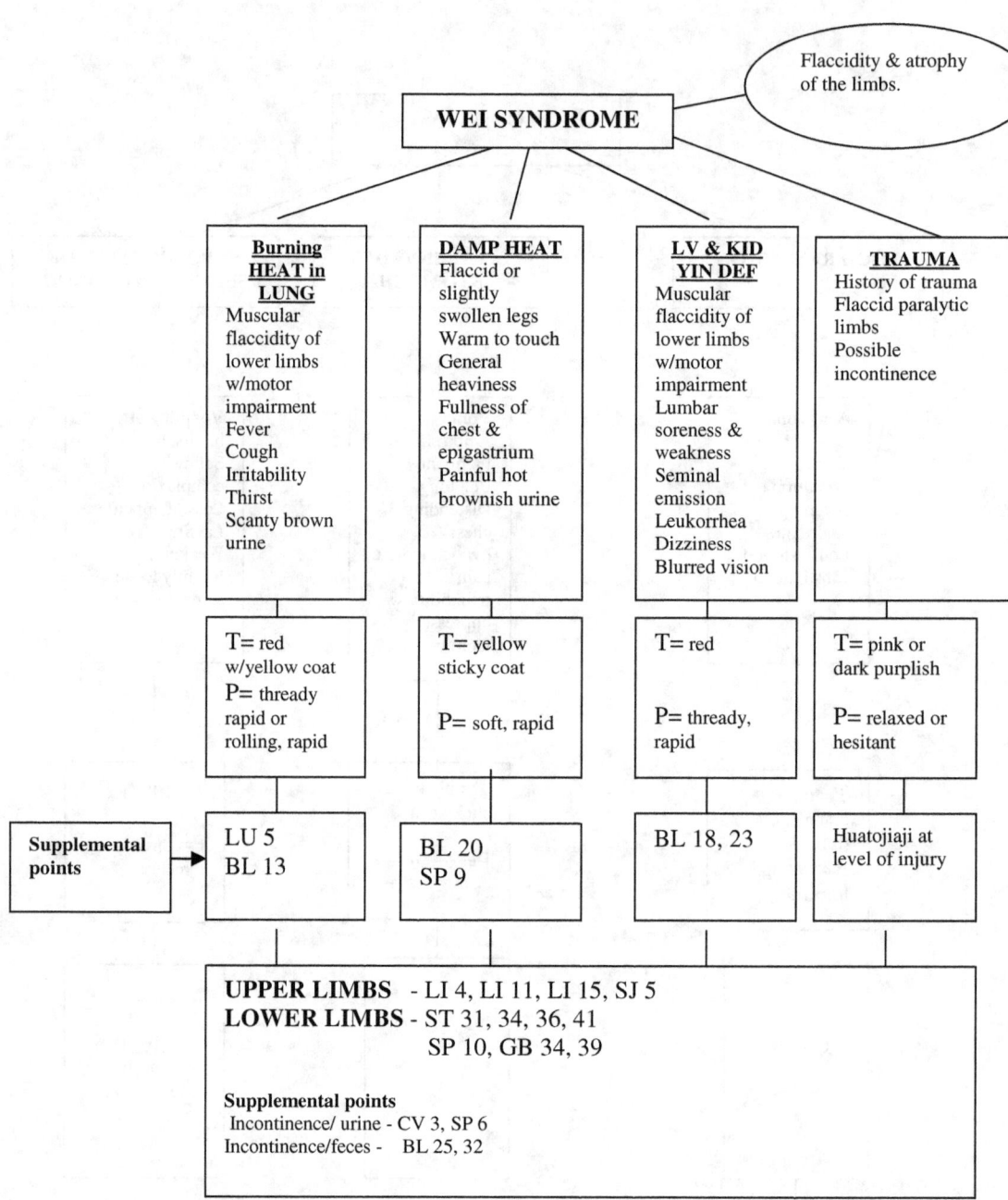

WEI SYNDROME

Flaccidity & atrophy of the limbs.

Burning HEAT in LUNG	**DAMP HEAT**	**LV & KID YIN DEF**	**TRAUMA**
Muscular flaccidity of lower limbs w/motor impairment Fever Cough Irritability Thirst Scanty brown urine	Flaccid or slightly swollen legs Warm to touch General heaviness Fullness of chest & epigastrium Painful hot brownish urine	Muscular flaccidity of lower limbs w/motor impairment Lumbar soreness & weakness Seminal emission Leukorrhea Dizziness Blurred vision	History of trauma Flaccid paralytic limbs Possible incontinence
T= red w/yellow coat P= thready rapid or rolling, rapid	T= yellow sticky coat P= soft, rapid	T= red P= thready, rapid	T= pink or dark purplish P= relaxed or hesitant
LU 5 BL 13	BL 20 SP 9	BL 18, 23	Huatojiaji at level of injury

Supplemental points →

UPPER LIMBS - LI 4, LI 11, LI 15, SJ 5
LOWER LIMBS - ST 31, 34, 36, 41
SP 10, GB 34, 39

Supplemental points
 Incontinence/ urine - CV 3, SP 6
Incontinence/feces -   BL 25, 32

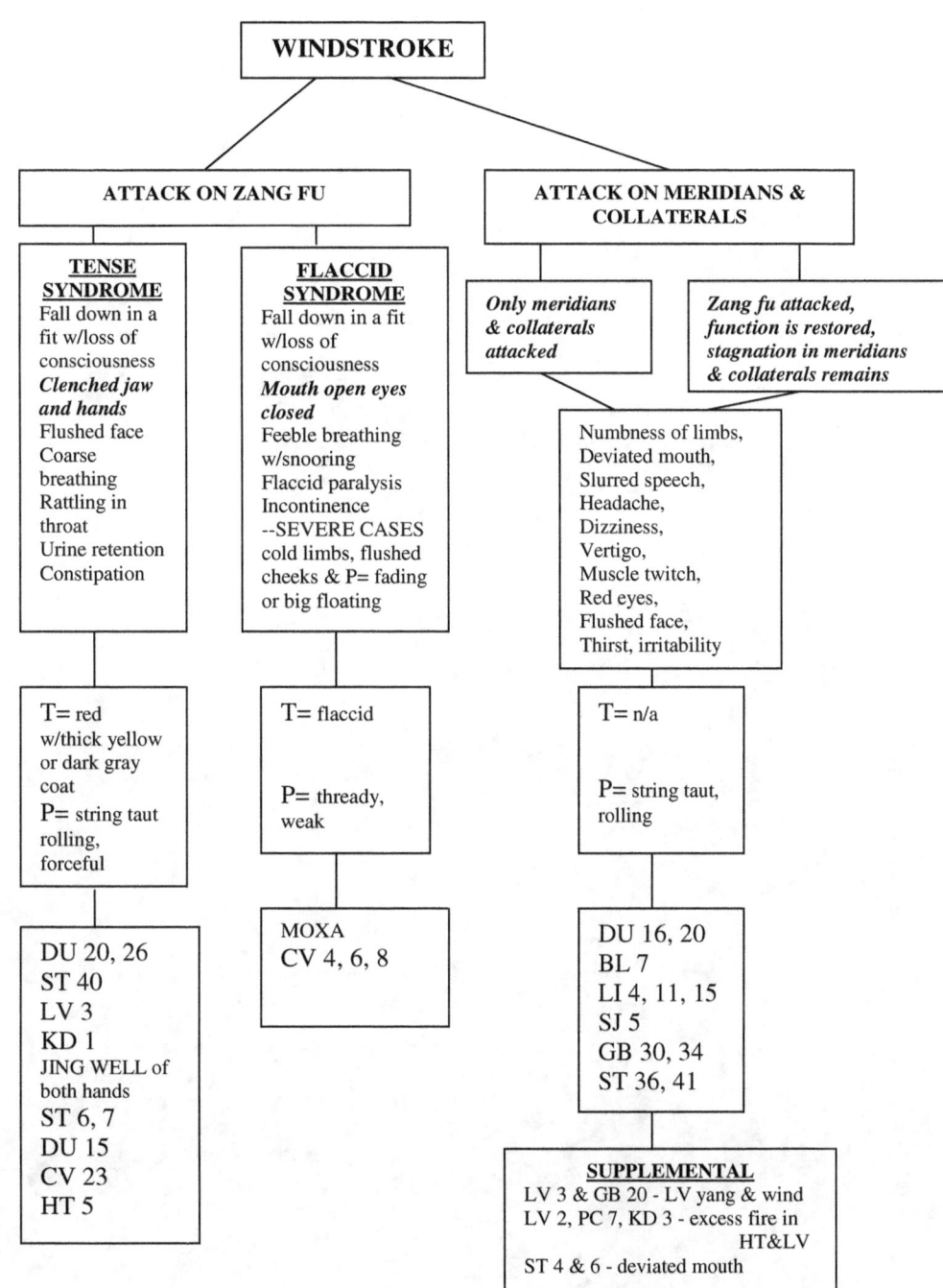

WINDSTROKE

ATTACK ON ZANG FU

TENSE SYNDROME
Fall down in a fit w/loss of consciousness
Clenched jaw and hands
Flushed face
Coarse breathing
Rattling in throat
Urine retention
Constipation

T= red w/thick yellow or dark gray coat
P= string taut rolling, forceful

DU 20, 26
ST 40
LV 3
KD 1
JING WELL of both hands
ST 6, 7
DU 15
CV 23
HT 5

FLACCID SYNDROME
Fall down in a fit w/loss of consciousness
Mouth open eyes closed
Feeble breathing w/snooring
Flaccid paralysis
Incontinence
--SEVERE CASES cold limbs, flushed cheeks & P= fading or big floating

T= flaccid

P= thready, weak

MOXA
CV 4, 6, 8

ATTACK ON MERIDIANS & COLLATERALS

Only meridians & collaterals attacked

Zang fu attacked, function is restored, stagnation in meridians & collaterals remains

Numbness of limbs,
Deviated mouth,
Slurred speech,
Headache,
Dizziness,
Vertigo,
Muscle twitch,
Red eyes,
Flushed face,
Thirst, irritability

T= n/a

P= string taut, rolling

DU 16, 20
BL 7
LI 4, 11, 15
SJ 5
GB 30, 34
ST 36, 41

SUPPLEMENTAL
LV 3 & GB 20 - LV yang & wind
LV 2, PC 7, KD 3 - excess fire in HT&LV
ST 4 & 6 - deviated mouth

ABDOMINAL DISTENSION EXCESS	CV12	ST36	ST25	ST37	LI 4	CV6	SP9
ABDOMINAL DISTENSION DEF	CV12	ST36	ST25	ST37	CV4	SP3	
ABDOMINAL PAIN (ACCUM OF COLD)	CV12	ST36	moxa CV8	SP4	LV13		
ABDOMINAL PAIN (DEF SPLEEN YANG)	CV12	ST36	CV6	BL 20,21	INNER NETTING		
ABDOMINAL PAIN (RETENTION OF FOOD)	CV12	ST36	CV6	ST25			
AMENORRHEA (BLOOD STAGNATION)	SP6	CV3	KD14	LI 4	LV3	SP10	ST29
AMENORRHEA (BLOOD DEPLETION)	SP6	CV4	ST36	BL18	BL20	BL23	
ASTHMA EXCESS WINDCOLD	BL13	BL12	DU14	LU7	LI 4		
ASTHMA EXCESS(RET OF PHLEG HEAT IN LU)	BL13	LU5	CV22	ST40	DINGCHUAN		
ASTHMA DEF LU DEFIC	BL13	LU9	SP3	ST36			
ASTHMA DEF KID DEF	BL13	KD3	BL23	CV6	CV17		
BI SYNDROME WANDERING	BL17	SP10					
BI SYNDROME PAINFUL	BL23	CV4					
BI SYNDROME FIXED	ST36	SP5					
BI SYNDROME HEAT	DU14	LI 11					
BOILS	DU10	DU12	PC4	LI 4	BL40		
BREAST ABSCESS	GB21	CV17	ST 18,36	SI 1	LV3		
COMMON COLD (WIND COLD)	LI 4	DU16	BL12	GB20	LU7		
COMMON COLD (WIND HEAT)	LI 4	DU14	LI 11	LU10	LU11	SJ5	
CONSTIPATION EXCESS HEAT	BL25	ST25	KD6	SJ6	LI 4	LI 11	
CONSTIPATION EXCESS QI STAG	BL25	ST25	KD6	SJ6	CV12	LV3	
CONSTIPATION DEFIC QI & BLOOD	BL25	ST25	KD6	SJ6	BL20	BL21	
CONSTIPATION DEFIC COLD	BL25	ST25	KD6	SJ6	moxa CV6	moxa CV8	ST36
COUGH (EPI) WIND COLD	BL13	LU7	LI 4	DU14	SJ5		
COUGH (EPI) WIND HEAT	BL13	LU7	LI 4	LU11			
COUGH (BLOCKAGE OF LU BY PHLEGM)	BL13	CV12	ST36	ST40			
COUGH (DRY LUNG DUE TO DEF YIN)	BL13	LU 1,6,7	KD6	BL17			

DEAFNESS & TINNITUS	EXCESS	LV/Gbfire	SJ 3,17	GB2	LV2	GB41			
DEAFNESS & TINNITUS	EXCESS	wind	SJ 3,17	GB2	SJ5	LI 4			
DEAFNESS & TINNITUS	DEF		SJ 3,17	GB2	BL23	DU4	KD3		
DEVIATION OF EYE & MOUTH			SJ17	GB14	TAIYANG	SI 18	ST4,6,7	LI 4	
DIARRHEA (ACUTE) COLD DAMP			ST36	ST25	moxa CV6	moxa CV12			
DIARRHEA (ACUTE) DAMP HEAT			ST36	ST25	ST44	SP9			
DIARRHEA (ACUTE) FOOD RET			ST36	ST25	INNER NEITING				
DIARRHEA (CHRONIC) DEF SPLN			ST36	BL20	LV13	SP3	CV12		
DIARRHEA (CHRONIC) DEF KID			ST36	BL20	BL23	KD3	moxa DU4	moxa CV4	
DIZZINESS (HYPERACTIVITY OF LV YANG)			GB20	BL18,23	KD3				
DIZZINESS (DEF OF QI/BLOOD)			BL20	CV4	DU20	ST36	SP6		
DIZZINESS (PHLEGM DAMP)			BL20	BL21	LV13	ST8	CV12	PC6	ST40
DYSENTERY	DAMP HEAT		ST25	ST37	LI 4, 11				
DYSENTERY	COLD DAMP		ST25	ST37	moxa CV6	moxa CV12	SP9		
DYSENTERY	FOOD RES		ST25	ST37	CV12	PC6			
DYSENTERY	INTERMITTENT		ST25	ST37	BL 20,21	CV4	ST36		
DYSMENORRHEA	EXCESS	lv qi stag	BL32	CV3	SP 8,10	LI 4	LV3		
DYSMENORRHEA	EXCESS	colddamp	BL32	CV3	SP 8,10	LI 4	LV3		
DYSMENORRHEA	DEF	qi / blood	CV4	BL 20,23	ST36	SP6			
DYSURIA CALCULI			BL28	CV3	BL39				
DYSURIA QI DYSF			BL28	CV3	LV2				
DYSURIA BLOOD IN URINE			BL28	CV3	SP 6,10				
DYSURIA MILKY URINE			BL28	CV3	BL23	KD6			
DYSURIA OVERSTRAIN			BL28	CV3	DU20	CV6	ST36		
EDEMA	YANG		LU7	LI 4, 6	SP9	BL39			
EDEMA	YIN		CV 4, 9	BL20	BL23	KD7	ST36		
EPIGASTRIC PAIN	RET OF FOOD		CV12	ST36	PC6	INNER NEITING			
EPIGASTRIC PAIN	LV INV SPL		CV12	ST36	PC6	LV 3, 14			
EPIGASTRIC PAIN	DEF ST W STAG OF COLD		CV12	ST36	PC6	CV6	SP4	BL20	

EPILEPSY	DURING	DU26	CV15	PC5	LV3	ST40	YINTANG
EPILEPSY	AFTER	BL15	HT 7	SP6	KD3	YAOQI	
EPISTAXIS	HEAT IN LU	LI 4	LI20	DU23			
EPISTAXIS	HEAT IN ST	LI 4	LI20	DU23	ST44		
EPISTAXIS	YIN DEF	LI 4	LI20	DU23	KD6		
ERYSIPELIS (HERPES ZOSTER) WIND HEAT		LI 4	LI 11	PC3	BL40	SP10	GB20
ERYSIPELIS (HERPES ZOSTER) DAMP HEAT		LI 4	LI 11	PC3	BL40	SP10	ST36
EYE PAIN CONGESTION,SWELLING	wind heat	BL1	GB20	LI 4	TAIYANG	LV2	SJ5
EYE PAIN CONGESTION,SWELLING	lv/gb fire	BL1	GB20	LI 4	TAIYANG	LV2	LV3
FACIAL PAIN	WIND COLD	GB20					
FACIAL PAIN	LV ST FIRE	LV3	ST44				
FACIAL PAIN	DEF YIN/EXC FIRE	SP6	KD6				
GOITER	Qi	SJ13	LI 4,17	SI 17	CV22	ST36	
GOITER	FLESH	SJ13	LI 4,17	SI 17	CV22	ST36	
HEADACHE (OCCIPITAL taiyang)		ST8	GB20	BL60	SI3	ST36	
HEADACHE (FRONTAL yangming)		ST8	DU23	LI 4	ST44	ST36	
HEADACHE (TEMPORAL shaoyang)		ST8	TAIYANG	GB8	SJ5	YINTANG	
HEADACHE (PARIETAL taiyang/jueyin)		DU20	SI3	BL67	LV3	GB41	
HEADACHE (LV FLAREUP)		DU20	GB5	GB20	LV3	LV2	
HEADACHE (DEF QI & BLOOD)		DU20	CV6	BL18,20,23	GB43	ST36	
HICCUPS RET OF FOOD		BL17	CV12	PC6	ST36	CV14	
HICCUPS QI STAG		BL17	CV12	PC6	ST36	CV17	LV3
HICCUPS COLD IN ST		BL17	CV12	PC6	ST36	CV13	
HYPOCHONDRIAC PAIN (EXCESS) qi stag		LV3	GB40				
HYPOCHONDRIAC PAIN (EXCESS) stag blood		BL18	BL17				
HYPOCHONDRIAC PAIN (DEFIC)		BL18	LV 3,14	BL23	SP6	ST36	
IMPOTENCE	DECL/MINGMEN	SP6	CV4	DU4	BL23	KD3	BL15
IMPOTENCE	DAMP HEAT	SP6	CV3	SP9	ST36		HT 7

Condition						HANDLING WELL PTS	
INFANTILE CONVULSIONS ACUTE wind heat	yintang	DU26	LV3	DU14	LI 11	LI 4	ST40
INFANTILE CONVULSIONS ACUTE phlegm heat	yintang	DU26	LV3	SJ18	CV12	KD1	
INFANTILE CONVULSIONS ACUTE sudden fright	yintang	DU26	LV3	sishencong	PC8	LV3	KD2
INFANTILE CONVULSIONS CHRONIC	DU 20,24	CV 4,6	ST36	BL 20,23	CV12		
INFANTILE DIARRHEA (OVERFEEDING)	SIFENG	ST25	ST37	CV6	CV11		
INFANTILE DIARRHEA (DAMP HEAT)	SIFENG	ST25	ST37	LI 4	LI 11		
INFANTILE MALNUTRITION (SP/ST DEFICIENCY)	SIFENG	CV10	BL 20,21	ST36	SP3	Baichongwo	
INFANTILE MALNUTRITION ((PARASITES)	SIFENG	CV10	BL 20,21	ST36	SP3		
INFANTILE PARALYSIS (UPPER LIMBS)	LI 4, 11	LI 15	DU14	BL10	SJ5		
INFANTILE PARALYSIS (LOWER LIMBS)	ST 31,36	ST41	GB 30,34	GB39	SP6	BL60	
INFANTILE PARALYSIS (ABDOMINAL MUSCLES)	ST 21,25	GB26	CV4	BL21			
INSOMNIA (HT & SP DEF)	HT 7	SP6	ANMIAN	BL15	BL20	moxa SP1	
INSOMNIA (HT & KD DISHARMONY)	HT 7	SP6	ANMIAN	BL15	BL23	KD3	
INSOMNIA (LIVER YANG RISING)	HT 7	SP6	ANMIAN	BL 18,19	GB12		
INSOMNIA (ST & SP DEFICIENCY)	HT 7	SP6	ANMIAN	BL21	ST36		
INSUFFICIENT LACTATION QI/BLD DEF	ST18	CV17	GB21	SI 1	BL20	ST36	SP6
INSUFFICIENT LACTATION LV QI STAG	ST18	CV17	GB21	SI 1	LV14	LV3	PC6
INTESTIONAL ABSCESS	ST 25,37	LI 11	LANWEI				
JAUNDICE (YANG/DAMP HEAT)	DU9	SP9	ST36	BL18,19	LV3	GB34	
JAUNDICE (YIN /COLD DAMP)	DU9	SP9	ST36	BL18,19	moxa BL20	moxa BL48	
LOW BACK PAIN COLDDAMP	BL23	DU3	BL40	BL 25, 26			
LOW BACK PAIN (KID DEF ESS)	BL23	DU3	BL40				
LOW BACK PAIN (KID DEF YANG)	BL23	DU3	BL40	DU4	YAOYAN		
LOW BACK PAIN (KID DEF YIN)	BL23	DU3	BL40	BL52	KD3		
LOW BACK PAIN (TRAUMATIC)	BL23	DU3	BL40	DU26	YAOTONGXUE		
MALARIA	DU 13,14	SI 3	PC5	SJ5	GB41		
MANIC DEPRESSIVE DEPRES	ST40	BL15	BL18	BL20	HT 7		
MANIC DEPRESSIVE MANIC	ST40	DU14	DU16	DU26	PC6		

MELANCHOLIA (CONSTR LV QI)		LV3	BL18	SP4	CV 12,17	ST36	
MELANCHOLIA (LV FIRE)		LV3	GB 34,43	CV13	SJ6	LV2	
MELANCHOLIA (PHLEGM STAG)		LV3	CV 17,22	PC6	ST40		
MELANCHOLIA (DEF BLOOD)(HYSTERIA)		LV3	CV14	HT 7	SP6		
MENSTRUATION	EARLY HEAT/BLOOD	LI 11	SP10	CV3	KD5		
MENSTRUATION	EARLY DEF SP QI	CV6	CV12	SP6	ST36		
MENSTRUATION	IRREG LV QI STAG	CV6	KD14	PC5	LV5		
MENSTRUATION	IRREG KID DEF	BL23	CV4	KD8			
MENSTRUATION	LATE IRREG DEF BLD	CV6	CV4	SP6			
MENSTRUATION	LATE IRREG COLD/BLD	CV6	CV4	SP6			
MENSTRUATION	LATE IRREG STAG QI	CV6	ST25	SP8	LV3		
MORBID LEUCORRHEA	SP DEF	GB26	CV6	BL30	SP9	ST36	
MORBID LEUCORRHEA	KD DEF	GB26	CV4	BL23	KD 7, 12		
MORBID LEUCORRHEA	DAMP HEAT	CV3	BL32	SP6	LV 3, 5	SP10	LI 11
MORNING SICKNESS	SP/ST DEF	CV12	ST36	PC6	CV13	SP4	
MORNING SICKNESS	LV INV ST	CV12	ST36	PC6	CV17	LV3	
MUMPS		SJ 5,17	ST6	LI 4,11			
NASAL DISCHARGE (RHINORRHEA)		LI 4	LI20	LU 7	BITONG	YINTANG	
NOCTURNAL ENURESIS		BL 23,28	CV3	SP6	LV1		
NOCTURNAL EMISSION		CV3	LV1	SP6	BL23	BL28	
OPTIC ATROPHY (DEF LV & KD YIN)		GB 20,39	BL1	QIUHOU			
OPTIC ATROPHY (DEF OF QI & BLOOD)		ST38	SP6				
OPTIC ATROPHY (STAG OF LV QI)		LV 3,14	GB34				
PALPITATIONS	MIND DISTRBD	BL15	CV14	HT 7	PC6	HT5	GB40
PALPITATIONS	DEF QI/BLOOD	BL15	CV14	HT 7	PC6	BL 20,21	ST36
PALPITATIONS	HT FIR/KD YIN DEF	BL15	CV14	HT 7	PC6	BL 14,23	KD3
PALPITATIONS	RET OF FLUID	BL15	CV14	HT 7	PC6	CV 4,8,9	SP9
PALPITATIONS	DEF SP/KD YANG	BL15	CV14	HT 7	PC6	CV 4,8,9	SP9

PROLAPSE OF RECTUM		DU1	DU20	ST36	BL25		
PROLONGED LABOR	QI & BLOOD DEF	BL67	SP6	ST36	ST36		
PROLONGED LABOR	QI & BLOOD STAG	BL67	SP6	LI 4			
SEMINAL EMISSION	NOCT EMISSION	HT 7	BL15	KD3	BL52	moxa CV6	
SEMINAL EMISSION	SPERMATORRHEA	BL23	SP6	KD12	moxa CV4		
SORE THROAT (EXCESS HEAT)		LI 4	LI 11	ST44	SI17		
SORE THROAT (KID YIN DEF)		LU 7,10	LI18	KD 3,6	CV23		
SPRAIN & CONTUSION		TREAT ASHI POINTS					
SUNSTROKE	MILD	BL40	DU14	LI 11	PC6	SHIXUAN	
SUNSTROKE	SEVERE	BL40	DU20	DU26	PC3		
SYNCOPE	DEF	DU26	DU20	PC6	CV6	ST36	
SYNCOPE	EXCESS	DU26	PC 8,9	LI 4	LV3	KD1	
TOOTHACHE	ST FIRE	ST6	ST7	LI 4	ST44		
TOOTHACHE	WIND FIRE	ST6	ST7	LI 4	SJ2	SJ5	GB20
TOOTHACHE	DEF KID	ST6	ST7	KD3			
TORTICOLLIS		DU14	BL10,60	SI 3,7,14	GB39	LU7	Laozhen
URINARY RETENTION	ACC/HEAT/BLAD	CV3	SP6	BL28	BL39		
URINARY RETENTION	dec/MINGMEN/FIRE	CV3	SP6	DU4	DU20	BL23	
URINARY RETENTION	DAMAGE OF QI	CV3	SP6	KD5	ST28		SJ4
UTERINE BLEEDING (EXC HEAT)		SP1	CV3	SP10	LV8	ST36	
UTERINE BLEEDING (QI DEF)		SP1	DU20	CV4	ST36	SP9	
UTERINE PROLAPSE (QI DEF)		DU20	CV6	CV12	ST36	ST29	
UTERINE PROLAPSE (KID DEF)		CV4	LV8	KD6	ZIGONG		SJ4
URTICARIA (WIND HEAT)		LI 4,11	BL40	SP 6,10	DU14		
URTICARIA (WIND DAMP)		LI 4,11	BL40	SP 6,10	SP9		
URTICARIA (ACCUM OF HEAT ST/INTE)		LI 4,11	BL40	SP 6,10	ST 25,36		

VOMITING (FOOD RETENTION)	CV12	ST36	SP4	PC6	CV10
VOMITING (LIVER INVADES STOMACH)	CV12	ST36	SP4	PC6	LV3
VOMITING (HYPOFXN SP/ST)	CV12	ST36	SP4	PC6	BL20	INNER NEITING

WEI SYNDROME (HEAT IN LUNG)	LU5	BL23	
WEI SYNDROME (DAMP HEAT)	BL20	SP9	
WEI SYNDROME (LV & KID YIN DEF)	BL18	BL23	
WEI SYNDROME (TRAUMA)	Huatojiaji at level of injury		

WINDSTROKE ZANGFU TENSE	DU20	DU26	ST40	LV3	KD1	JINGWELL/HANDS
WINDSTROKE ZANGFU FLACCID	moxa CV 4,6,8			
WINDSTROKE ATTK ON COLL/MERID	DU20	DU16	BL7	LI 4,11,15	SJ5	GB 30,34 ST 36,41

INDEX

A

B

C

D

S

T

U

V

W

Notes

Notes

Notes

www.ingramcontent.com/pod-product-compliance
Lightning Source LLC
Chambersburg PA
CBHW081140170526
45165CB00008B/2747